# C

The Most Powerful Tool To ~~ Obesity

**DR. PETER HAWKINS**

All rights reserved. No part of this publication may be reproduced, distributed or transmitted in any form or by any means, including photocopying, recording or other electronic or mechanical methods, without the prior written permission of the publisher, except in the case of brief quotations embodied in critical reviews and certain other noncommercial uses permitted by copyright law.

Copyright © 2024  DR. PETER HAWKINS

# TABLE OF CONTENTS

Introduction

1.1 Overview of Contrave
1.2 Purpose and Benefits
Composition

2.1 Active Ingredients
2.2 Inactive Ingredients
Mechanism of Action

3.1 How Contrave Works
3.2 Targeted Areas in the Body
Indications

4.1 Approved Medical Uses
4.2 Patient Eligibility Criteria
Dosage and Administration

5.1 Recommended Dosage
5.2 Administration Guidelines
Clinical Trials

6.1 Efficacy Studies
6.2 Safety and Tolerability

Side Effects

7.1 Common Adverse Reactions
7.2 Serious Side Effects
Contraindications

8.1 Conditions Where Contrave is Not Recommended
8.2 Drug Interactions
Warnings and Precautions

9.1 Special Considerations
9.2 Monitoring Requirements
Patient Counseling

10.1 Guidance for Patients
10.2 Lifestyle Recommendations
Frequently Asked Questions (FAQs)
Conclusion

# INTRODUCTION

A prescription drug called Contrave helps people control their weight by targeting the neurological and physiological elements of hunger regulation. Contrave, which was first brought to the market as a blend of two different medications bupropion and naltrexone offers a special method of managing weight.

The antidepressant and smoking cessation medication bupropion acts on the brain's neurotransmitters, mainly dopamine and norepinephrine. In addition to being essential for mood regulation, these neurotransmitters have an impact on appetite and food desires, which is vital to managing weight. Bupropion helps decrease appetite and may lessen the impulse to overeat by modifying these substances.

The second ingredient in Contrave, naltrexone, has long been used to treat alcohol and narcotic addictions. The function of naltrexone in Contrave is complex. It is thought to affect the reward system connected to food consumption, which may lessen the enjoyable feelings connected to eating. Additionally, by affecting endorphins and other neurotransmitters, naltrexone may indirectly affect behavior related to food.

The goal of combining these two drugs in Contrave is to offer a complete weight-management solution. Contrave aims to address the complicated nature of obesity by addressing both the psychological aspects of appetite and the neural circuits involved in reward and craving. It is noteworthy that a full weight loss program consisting of dietary adjustments, increased physical activity, and behavioral counseling is usually recommended in addition to Contrave prescriptions.

Clinical trials have investigated Contrave's safety and effectiveness in a range of populations. According to the results, people who use Contrave in addition to making lifestyle changes may lose more weight than those who only make lifestyle changes. Contrave does have certain possible adverse effects and contraindications, just like any drug. Individuals who are thinking about using Contrave should have in-depth conversations with medical professionals to determine whether it is appropriate for their unique set of circumstances.

By combining naltrexone and bupropion to address the neurological and psychological elements of hunger regulation, Contrave offers a fresh strategy to weight management. Its function in all-inclusive weight-loss plans emphasizes the significance of a diverse strategy in the fight against obesity. As with any drug, people should use Contrave under the supervision of healthcare professionals and with a thorough awareness of its mechanisms, potential benefits, and related issues.

# PURPOSE AND BENEFITS

Contrave is primarily intended to help people manage their weight by providing a pharmaceutical intervention to support lifestyle changes. By targeting numerous issues linked with obesity, such as appetite control, cravings, and the neurological circuits related to food reward, Contrave's main goal is to aid in weight loss.

Contrave has advantages that go beyond the conventional strategy of only reducing hunger. Its special blend of naltrexone and bupropion takes advantage of these drugs' synergistic effects to address both the neurological and psychological components of weight regulation. Bupropion, well-known for helping people quit smoking and treating depression, suppresses appetite by modifying neurotransmitters including dopamine and norepinephrine. Consequently, there may be a decrease in food cravings and the impulse to overindulge.

Naltrexone adds a unique component to Contrave's mechanism of action. Naltrexone was first used to treat opiate and alcohol dependency. Naltrexone works by altering the brain's reward system, which reduces the feelings of pleasure that come with eating. Contrave's dual-action technique sets it apart from other weight-loss pills and highlights its all-encompassing approach to addressing the complex nature of obesity.

The possibility for increased weight loss when Contrave is used in conjunction with lifestyle changes is one of the main advantages seen in clinical trials. Patients who use Contrave together with food modifications, increased exercise, and behavioral counseling have lost significantly more weight than those who only made lifestyle changes. This emphasizes Contrave's function in a comprehensive weight-management program where medication supports and enhances healthy lifestyle changes.

Moreover, using Contrave for purposes other than weight loss is possible. Its possible effects on metabolic markers, such as enhanced lipid profiles and insulin sensitivity, have been the subject of some research. The overall good health effects of using Contrave are facilitated by these extra metabolic advantages.

It is critical to understand that Contrave is not a one-size-fits-all treatment, even though it may have certain advantages. Since each person's reaction to a medication is different, medical practitioners should carefully consider factors such medical history, current conditions, and potential drug interactions. Patients and their healthcare providers should consult together to decide whether to use Contrave, assessing the possible advantages against any potential hazards.

Contrave's main goal is to support weight management by using a thorough strategy that takes into account the neurological and psychological aspects of obesity. Its advantages include suppressing hunger, possibly improving metabolic parameters, and having the ability to facilitate weight loss when combined with more comprehensive lifestyle adjustment programs. To maximize the advantages of Contrave, like with any drug, educated decision-making in cooperation with medical specialists is essential.

# ACTIVE INGREDIENTS

Bupropion and naltrexone work together to provide the pharmacological effect of Contrave, a prescription drug intended to help with weight management. Together, these components make a unique blend that addresses many facets of the body's physiology and neurochemistry, which enhances its ability to aid in weight loss. Here, we explore the intricacies of these active components, looking at their unique characteristics, modes of action, and combined effects that make Contrave what it is.

- **Bupropion:** A major ingredient of Contrave is bupropion, an atypical antidepressant and smoking cessation medication. It is included in this weight-loss drug because of its effects on brain neurotransmitters, especially dopamine and norepinephrine. The main way that bupropion works is by preventing these neurotransmitters from being reabsorbed, which raises their concentrations in the synaptic cleft.
- **Modulation of Neurotransmitters:** The stress hormone and neurotransmitter

norepinephrine is essential to the body's "fight or flight" reaction. Bupropion regulates arousal, attention, and, crucially, appetite by adjusting norepinephrine levels. Often referred to as the "feel-good" neurotransmitter, dopamine plays a role in reward-motivated behavior, which includes the enjoyment that comes from eating.

One theory is that bupropion suppresses hunger by acting on these neurotransmitters. It may lessen cravings for food and sensations of hunger by raising norepinephrine and dopamine levels, which would ultimately help create a caloric deficit and aid in weight loss.

- **Quitting Smoking Attributes:** Bupropion was first created as a smoking cessation tool, but it soon became known for its capacity to lessen withdrawal symptoms and cravings for nicotine. This is significant in the context of Contrave because it points to a potential bonus for those with co-occurring conditions like smoking, where weight gain is a common worry when quitting.
- **Prolonged-Release Mixture:** Bupropion is frequently used in the Contrave formulation

in an extended-release form. This makes it possible for the drug to be released gradually over time, affecting neurotransmitter levels more continuously and maybe increasing the medicine's ability to regulate hunger.
- **naltrexone:** Naltrexone, the second active component in Contrave, is an opioid receptor antagonist. The addition of naltrexone to Contrave adds a special touch to the weight-management mix. Naltrexone has long been utilized in the treatment of opiate and alcohol addictions.
- **Opioid Receptor Resistant Abuse:** In order to prevent endorphins and exogenous opioids from attaching to opioid receptors, naltrexone works by opposing these receptors. The function of endorphins in the brain's reward system especially in reaction to pleasurable stimuli like food makes this action important for managing weight.
- **Impact on Food Reward Routes:** The pleasure and reinforcement that come with some behaviors, like eating, are closely tied to the reward system, which is controlled by neurotransmitters like dopamine. The opioid receptor antagonism of naltrexone is expected

to lessen the rewarding effects of eating, which may lessen the reinforcement that encourages overindulgence in food and poor eating habits.
- **Effect on Wants:** Naltrexone has potential impacts on food cravings in addition to its effects on the reward system. By interfering with the neurochemical mechanisms linked to cravings, it advances the general objective of suppressing hunger and enhancing self-control over food consumption.
- **Combinatorial Impacts in Contrave:** Contrave's bupropion and naltrexone combo works synergistically rather than just additively. The two components work in tandem to address distinct aspects of the intricate relationship between behavior, appetite regulation, and neurochemistry.
- **Entire Appetite Management:** While naltrexone works on a separate axis by altering the reward system, bupropion reduces appetite and cravings primarily by targeting neurotransmitters like norepinephrine and dopamine. When combined, these effects provide a more all-encompassing approach to hunger regulation,

possibly producing a stronger result than when one ingredient is used alone.
- **Possibility of Increased Loss of Weight:** Clinical research have indicated that as compared to monotherapies or lifestyle changes alone, the combination of bupropion and naltrexone in Contrave may result in greater weight loss. This emphasizes the value of a multimodal strategy for managing weight, in which medication therapies support and enhance healthy lifestyle adjustments.
- **Clinical Trials and Evidence:** Many clinical trials have been conducted to evaluate the safety and effectiveness of Contrave, which is derived from the combination of naltrexone and bupropion. These clinical trials encompass a range of patient demographics and assess multiple factors, such as reduction in body weight, alterations in metabolic indicators, and the medication's general acceptability.
- **Results of Weight Loss:** According to clinical research, people who used Contrave in addition to making lifestyle changes lost more weight than those who only made

lifestyle changes. The fact that this weight loss was frequently maintained over a longer time frame highlights how long-lasting Contrave's benefits are in aiding continued weight management attempts.
- **Impact on Metabolism:** Contrave has been studied for its possible effects on metabolic parameters in addition to weight loss. Studies have shown improvements in lipid profiles and insulin sensitivity, suggesting that the drug has wider metabolic advantages. These results advance our knowledge of Contrave as a medicine that does more than just decrease hunger.
- **Tolerance and Safety:** The safety profile of Contrave is important to take into account, just like it is with other drug. Clinical trials evaluate general tolerability, possible drug interactions, and the incidence of side events. Although headaches, nausea, and constipation are common side effects, major adverse events are very uncommon.

Bupropion and naltrexone, the active components of Contrave, combine to offer a special and all-encompassing method of weight management. The reduction of appetite is facilitated by bupropion's control over neurotransmitters, and the medication's effectiveness is further enhanced by naltrexone's effects on cravings and the reward system. The combination of these ingredients, backed by a wealth of clinical data, emphasizes Contrave's potential as a useful tool for tackling the intricate and multidimensional aspects of obesity. Like with any drug, those who are thinking about using Contrave should have educated conversations with medical specialists to determine whether it is appropriate for their particular set of circumstances and to maximize the potential advantages while limiting the risks.

# INACTIVE INGREDIENTS

In addition to bupropion and naltrexone, the active ingredients in Contrave, a drug intended to help with weight management, also comprise a number of inactive chemicals that support the drug's overall formulation, stability, and bioavailability. In this investigation, we go into great length on the inactive components of Contrave, learning about their functions, possible side effects, and the factors that went into choosing them for the recipe.

**The Function of Inactive Substances**

Excipients, sometimes referred to as inactive ingredients, are components of a drug's formulation that fulfill a number of necessary purposes but do not add to the drug's therapeutic benefits. These include boosting stability, easing the release of the drug, enhancing taste or appearance, and guaranteeing the medication's general safety and efficacy. When it comes to Contrave, the inactive elements are essential to the distribution and functionality of the active substances.

- **Ingredients for Contrave:** A range of inactive components, each selected for their distinct qualities and contributions to the overall features of the medication, may be included in the particular formulation of Contrave. We can examine broad types of inactive chemicals prevalent in many medicinal formulations, even though the exact composition is private.

**1. binders:** Substances known as binders aid in keeping the medication's active and inactive ingredients together. They aid in the cohesive tablet or capsule's development. Polyvinylpyrrolidone, starches, and derivatives of cellulose are common binders.

**2. Diluents or Fillers:** In order to ensure that each tablet or capsule contains a consistent amount of the active ingredient, fillers or diluents are added to enhance the bulk of the medication. Lactose, microcrystalline cellulose, and calcium phosphate are a few examples.

**3. Breakers:** Disintegrants help release the active components for absorption by encouraging the tablet or capsule to break apart in the gastrointestinal system. Cross-linked polyvinylpyrrolidone and croscarmellose sodium are common disintegrants.

4. **Gliders:** During the manufacturing process, glideants enhance the powder mixture's flow

characteristics, guaranteeing consistent tablet or capsule formation. Glidants include talc and colloidal silicon dioxide.

**5. Coating Substances:** Coating agents have a number of functions, such as preventing the active components from degrading, hiding taste, and making the product easier to swallow. Polymers like polyethylene glycol and hydroxypropyl methylcellulose can be used as coating materials.

**6. Coloring Materials:** To improve the medication's look and make it more recognizable to patients and healthcare providers, coloring additives are added. They could consist of artificial or natural coloring agents.

**7. Agents of Flavor:** To enhance patients' taste and palatability, flavoring compounds may be used into certain formulations, particularly those intended as orally disintegrating pills or liquids.

**8. Preservatives:** Contrave is usually administered orally in a solid dose form, however in some formulations like liquid suspensions preservatives may be added to stop microbiological growth and preserve product stability.

- **Taking Into Account Inactive Ingredients:** Like any drug, Contrave's inactive ingredient composition and selection are subject to stringent regulatory criteria and scrutiny. The choice of excipients is influenced by a number of criteria, including as stability, manufacturability, compatibility with the active components, and the intended release profile.

**1. Harmony:** For the medication to be stable and effective, the inactive ingredients must work well with the active ingredients. When developing a formulation, interactions between active and inactive ingredients are carefully considered.

**2. Producability:** The excipients selected should make production easier and provide consistency and repeatability in the creation of the finished dosage form. For effective production, excipients that support the granulation, compression, and coating processes are essential.

**3. Consistency:** Stability tests are carried out to evaluate the medication's long-term stability while taking humidity, temperature, and light exposure into account. The formulation's overall stability is aided by inactive components.

**4. Profile of Release:** The selection of inactive components, especially disintegrants and coatings,

affects the release profile of the active compounds. Whether the medicine has an immediate or prolonged release depends on these factors.
- **Possible Things to Think About for Patients:** Despite the fact that inert substances are usually thought to be harmless, it's crucial that patients and medical professionals are aware of their existence. Certain excipients may cause allergies or sensitivities in certain people. For instance, people who are lactose intolerant should exercise caution because lactose is frequently used as a filler in pharmaceuticals.

Alternative formulations or drugs may be taken into consideration in circumstances when patients have known sensitivities or allergies to specific inactive components. When assessing a patient's medical history and recommending medications that are in line with specific health needs, healthcare practitioners are essential.

The inactive components of Contrave make a substantial contribution to the drug's overall composition and effectiveness. Although these constituents might not have a direct impact on the therapeutic outcomes, they are essential for maintaining stability, manufacturing viability, and patient acceptance. Excipients are chosen with great care to ensure that the medication is safe and effective while also meeting regulatory requirements. It is recommended that patients tell healthcare practitioners of any allergies or sensitivities so that tailored drug management strategies can be implemented.

# HOW CONTRAVE WORKS

The weight-management medicine Contrave, which is prescribed, functions by a complex mechanism involving its two active components, naltrexone and bupropion. Investigating each of these components' separate functions as well as the synergistic effects they produce when combined is necessary to comprehend how Contrave functions. This thorough analysis sheds light on the behavioral, physiological, and neurochemical mechanisms underlying Contrave's effects on hunger control and weight loss.

**The Function of Bupropion:**

**1. Modulation of Neurotransmitters:** Basic properties of bupropion include being an aminoketone class antidepressant. Its main mode of action is the suppression of neurotransmitter reuptake, specifically dopamine and norepinephrine. The stress hormone and neurotransmitter norepinephrine is essential to the body's fight-or-flight reaction. Elevated arousal and attentiveness can be attributed to elevated norepinephrine levels.

Dopamine is linked to behavior that is driven by rewards; it is sometimes referred to as the "feel-good" neurotransmitter. The brain's pleasure and reward system is thought to be impacted by bupropion's effects on dopamine levels.

**2. Suppression of Appetite:** An appetite suppressant effect of bupropion is thought to arise from its regulation of dopamine and norepinephrine. It might lessen cravings for overindulging and sensations of hunger by affecting these neurotransmitters.

The impact on appetite regulation helps create the calorie shortfall required for weight loss. People who use Contrave may notice a decrease in their appetites for food and an improvement in their ability to control portion sizes.

**3. Quitting Smoking Attributes:** Bupropion was first created as a smoking cessation tool, but it soon became known for its capacity to lessen withdrawal symptoms and cravings for nicotine.

This point is pertinent to the discussion of Contrave because it raises the possibility of an extra advantage for those who have co-occurring conditions like smoking, where weight gain is a common worry when quitting.

4. **Prolonged-Release Mixture:** Bupropion is frequently included in Contrave in an extended-release formulation. Because of the formulation's ability to deliver the medication gradually, neurotransmitter levels can be continuously affected. An other factor in the medicine's ability to support long-term weight management attempts is its extended-release characteristic.

**The Function of Naltrexone:**

**1. Opioid Receptor Resistant Abuse:** The second active component in Contrave, naltrexone, is an antagonist of opioid receptors. It functions by preventing endorphins and exogenous opioids from attaching themselves to opioid receptors.

Because endorphins are engaged in the brain's reward system, especially in reaction to pleasurable stimuli like food, this action is important when it comes to managing weight.

**2. Impact on Food Reward Routes:** The pleasurable effects of eating are hypothesized to be mitigated by naltrexone's opioid receptor antagonism. Overeating and poor eating patterns may be lessened by interfering with the neurochemical mechanisms linked to the reward system.

A shift in the psychological reaction to food is brought about by the influence on food reward circuits, which may lessen the enjoyment that comes from eating.

**3. Effect on Wants:** Naltrexone has potential impacts on food cravings in addition to its effects on the reward system. By interfering with the neurochemical mechanisms linked to cravings, it advances the general objective of suppressing hunger and enhancing self-control over food consumption.

This is especially important for people who have trouble with emotional or craving-driven eating habits.

**Combinatorial Impacts in Contrave:**

**1. Entire Appetite Management:** The synergistic action of bupropion and naltrexone together is produced by Contrave. While naltrexone works on a separate axis by altering the reward system, bupropion reduces appetite and cravings primarily by targeting neurotransmitters like norepinephrine and dopamine.

When combined, these effects provide a more all-encompassing approach to hunger regulation, possibly producing a stronger result than when one ingredient is used alone.

**2. Possibility of Increased Loss of Weight:** Clinical research have indicated that as compared to monotherapies or lifestyle changes alone, the combination of bupropion and naltrexone in Contrave may result in greater weight loss.

This emphasizes the value of a multimodal strategy for managing weight, in which medication therapies support and enhance healthy lifestyle adjustments.

**3. Effect on Behavior:** Contrave has behavioral effects in addition to its neurochemical ones. Eating behavior and patterns may change as a result of the modification of the reward and reinforcement dynamics linked to food.

One important component of Contrave's all-encompassing approach to weight management is the possibility of behavioral modifications.

**Clinical Trials and Evidence:**

**1. Results of Weight Loss:** According to clinical research, people who used Contrave in addition to making lifestyle changes lost more weight than those who only made lifestyle changes.

The fact that this weight loss was frequently maintained over a longer time frame highlights how long-lasting Contrave's benefits are in aiding continued weight management attempts.

**2. Impact on Metabolism:** The possible effects of contrave on metabolic parameters have been studied. Studies have shown improvements in lipid profiles and insulin sensitivity, suggesting that the drug has wider metabolic advantages.

The overall good health effects of using Contrave are facilitated by these extra metabolic advantages.

**3. Tolerance and Safety:** The safety profile of Contrave is important to take into account, just like it is with other drug. Clinical trials evaluate general tolerability, possible drug interactions, and the incidence of side events.

Although headaches, nausea, and constipation are common side effects, major adverse events are very uncommon.

Bupropion and naltrexone, the two active chemicals in Contrave, work together to provide a complex mechanism of action. The reduction of appetite is facilitated by bupropion's control over neurotransmitters, and the medication's effectiveness is further enhanced by naltrexone's effects on cravings and the reward system. These elements work together to provide a holistic approach to weight management that takes behavioral and physiological factors into account. Clinical research backs up Contrave's usefulness as an obesity prevention tool, giving users a variety of options for achieving and maintaining weight loss. Like with any drug, those who are thinking about using Contrave should have educated conversations with medical specialists to determine whether it is appropriate for their particular set of circumstances and to maximize the potential advantages while limiting the risks.

# TARGETED AREAS IN THE BODY

Bupropion and naltrexone, the main chemicals in Contrave, are a drug that helps with weight management. Contrave works by acting on specific parts of the body. This in-depth investigation explores the physiological and neurochemical dimensions of Contrave's effects, scrutinizing the particular bodily regions and systems that are pivotal to its mode of action.

**1. The CNS (central nervous system):**

**a. Modulation of Neurotransmitters:** Contrave's method of action primarily targets the central nervous system (CNS). One of Contrave's active chemicals, bupropion, affects the brain's neurotransmitters, especially dopamine and norepinephrine.

The stress response and arousal of the body are influenced by norepinephrine. Bupropion increases alertness and concentration via affecting norepinephrine levels.

One neurotransmitter linked to behavior driven by rewards is dopamine. Bupropion's impacts on dopamine levels may have an effect on the brain's pleasure and reward system, which could lessen the positive benefits of eating.

**b. Control of Appetite:** It's thought that bupropion suppresses hunger through altering neurotransmitters. It may lessen sensations of hunger and the impulse to overeat by affecting dopamine and norepinephrine levels.

The central nervous system (CNS) is involved in appetite regulation, and Contrave's actions support this process in its entirety.

## 2. The Endocrine System

**a. Control of Hormones:** The pituitary and hypothalamus are two examples of glands that are part of the endocrine system, which is responsible for controlling hormones that affect hunger and metabolism.

The effects of contrave on CNS neurotransmitters can affect hormonal signaling and lead to modifications in the levels of hormones that control appetite, including ghrelin and leptin.

**b. Metabolic Coefficients:** Metabolic control is intimately associated with the endocrine system. The possible effects of contrave on metabolic markers, such as enhanced insulin sensitivity, have been studied.

The combined effects of bupropion and naltrexone may improve metabolic indicators and improve the overall metabolic profile of Contrave users.

### 3. The digestive system

**a. Distribution and Absorption:** Contrave interacts with the gastrointestinal (GI) system during absorption and distribution, even though its main mechanisms of action are in the CNS and endocrine system.

One of the most important steps in releasing the active ingredients of Contrave for systemic circulation is their absorption in the gastrointestinal tract.

**b. Possible Impacts on the Absorption of Nutrients:** Although controlling appetite is the main goal of Contrave, it's important to take into account any possible impacts on nutrient absorption.

The GI system's reaction to the medicine may have an indirect effect on the absorption of nutrients, thus medical practitioners should take into account the general nutritional state of people taking Contrave.

### 4. Fat Cells in Adipose Tissue:

**a. Fat Metabolism:** Controlling lipid metabolism is essential for maintaining a healthy weight, especially in adipose tissue (fat cells).

Changes in lipid metabolism and the accumulation and use of fat may result from the effects of contrave on neurotransmitters and the central nervous system.

**b. Modifications to Body Composition:** Studies and clinical trials on Contrave have looked at how it affects lean and fat body mass as well as changes in body composition.

The medication's ability to modify adipose tissue is one of the ways it helps people undergoing weight control alter their body composition.

**5. Brain Circuitry and the Reward System:**

**a. Opioid Receptor Resistant Abuse:**
The second active component in Contrave, naltrexone, works by opposing opioid receptors. This process takes place in the brain's reward system, namely in the circuits linked to reinforcement and pleasure.

It is believed that the opioid receptor antagonistic effect lessens the pleasurable consequences of eating, which may lessen the reinforcement that encourages overindulgence in food.

**b. Modifications in Behavior:** One of the most important mechanisms influencing behavior, including eating behavior, is the reward system and related brain circuits.

Beyond just altering neurochemistry, contrast has a profound effect on the reward system, affecting behavior and possibly even changing eating habits.

**6. Heart System:**

**a. Heart-related Safety:** Given that obesity is frequently linked to cardiovascular risk factors, the cardiovascular system must be taken into account when using Contrave.

Clinical trials and post-marketing surveillance evaluate Contrave's cardiovascular safety by taking heart rate and blood pressure into account.

**b. Possible Impacts on Heart and Vascular Health:** Although controlling weight is Contrave's main goal, its impacts on metabolism and neurochemistry may also indirectly affect cardiovascular health.

Overall cardiovascular health may benefit from the medication's possible benefits in improving metabolic parameters.

### 7. Excretion and the Kidneys:

**a. Renal Clearance:** Medication excretion from the body is aided by the kidneys. The active components in Contrave are eliminated in part due to renal clearance.

Determining the proper dosage and evaluating the safety of the medicine require an understanding of the excretion mechanisms.

### 8. Metabolism and the Liver:

**a. The Metabolism of the Liver:** The active components in Contrave may be metabolized by the liver, which is an important organ in the metabolism of drugs.

When deciding whether or not to provide Contrave to people with liver diseases, it is important to take their function into account.

**b. Interactions between drugs:** One crucial factor to take into account when using Contrave is the possibility of drug interactions, especially when it comes to hepatic metabolism.

Medical practitioners assess potential drug interactions with other drugs that could impact the hepatic enzymes responsible for drug metabolism.

Contrave affects a number of specific physiological systems, including the liver, kidneys, endocrine system, gastrointestinal tract, adipose tissue, reward system, cardiovascular system, and central nervous system. Its active components, naltrexone and bupropion, interact intricately to produce a multidimensional weight-management strategy. Examining Contrave's effects on neurochemistry, behavior, metabolism, and other physiological systems is essential to understanding how it functions. Like with any drug, those who are thinking about using Contrave should have educated conversations with medical specialists to determine whether it is appropriate for their particular set of circumstances and to maximize the potential advantages while limiting the risks.

# APPROVED MEDICAL USES

Because bupropion and naltrexone are the only two active ingredients in Contrave, a prescription drug intended for weight control, it has certain approved medical applications. In-depth research on Contrave's medical uses, indications, and approved applications gives readers a thorough grasp of the medication's potential to treat obesity and related disorders.

**1. Handling Obesity:**

**a. BMI (body mass index) standards:** Adult obesity is recommended to be managed with Contrave. Body mass index (BMI), a metric derived from a person's weight and height, is frequently used to inform the decision to take Contrave.

The BMI requirements for prescription Contrave can vary, but in general, people with a BMI of 30 kg/m² or above or those with a BMI of 27 kg/m² or higher in the event of weight-related comorbidities are given consideration.

**b. Multidimensional Strategy:** Contrave is a component of a thorough, multidimensional weight-management strategy. This strategy incorporates behavioral therapy, dietary adjustments, and increased physical exercise.

The medicine is meant to be used in conjunction with a more comprehensive plan that aims to achieve and sustain weight loss, rather than as a stand-alone treatment.

**2. Comorbidities Related to Weight:**

**a. Diabetes Mellitus Type 2:** Type 2 diabetes mellitus is frequently linked to an elevated risk of obesity. For obese people with type 2 diabetes or those who are at risk of getting the disease, contrave may be taken into consideration.

Insulin sensitivity and glycemic control may both improve with weight loss from Contrave usage.

**b. dyslipidemia:** Obesity and dyslipidemia are frequently associated conditions that are defined by abnormal blood lipid levels. Those who have dyslipidemia and obesity may be offered Contrave.

Research indicates that improvements in lipid profiles might be attributed to Contrave's impact on lipid metabolism.

**c. High blood pressure:** One important risk factor for hypertension, or high blood pressure, is obesity.

For those who are obese and have high blood pressure, Contrave may be taken into consideration. Blood pressure decreases may be a result of weight loss with Contrave.

**3. Reducing Cardiovascular Risk:**

**a. Evaluation of Cardiovascular Risk:** In order to lower overall cardiovascular risk, contrave may be administered in the context of managing obesity. Healthcare providers evaluate each patient's unique cardiovascular risk factors while deciding whether or not to prescribe Contrave.

**4. Quitting Smoking in Obese Smokers:**

**a. Two Benefits of Quitting Smoking:** One of Contrave's main chemicals, bupropion, was first created as a smoking cessation tool.
Contrave's dual action addressing weight control and quitting smoking may be helpful for obese smokers.

**5. Selection Criteria for Patients:**

**a. Entire Assessment:** When deciding whether to administer Contrave, a thorough assessment of the patient's health history, present condition, and risk factors is conducted.

Healthcare providers take into account things like pre-existing medical issues, drug interactions, and the patient's capacity to follow through on lifestyle changes.

**b. Making Well-Informed Decisions:** A crucial component of the authorized medical uses of Contrave is informed decision-making. Patients receive information regarding the medicine, including possible advantages, side effects, and the significance of changing one's lifestyle.

This method guarantees that people actively participate in the decision-making process and are aware of Contrave's place in their overall weight-management strategy.

## 6. Treatment Duration:

**a. Extended-Term Administration:** Contrave isn't meant to be used temporarily; it's meant to be used for long-term weight management. Based on the patient's response to the drug, compliance with lifestyle changes, and continuous evaluation of benefits and hazards, the length of treatment is customized.

Whether or not to continue Contrave is determined by regular evaluations and ongoing monitoring.

**b. Considerations for Discontinuation:** If, after a given length of treatment, patients do not lose a specific amount of weight, stopping Contrave should be a consideration.

Other considerations that may influence the decision to stop taking Contrave include adverse effects, noncompliance, or modifications in the patient's condition.

**7. Counseling and Education for Patients:**

**a. All-encompassing Method:** One essential aspect of Contrave's authorized medical applications is patient education. People are informed about the drug, how it works, any possible adverse effects, and how important it is to change one's lifestyle.

The combined effects of counseling on food modifications, increased exercise, and behavioral techniques improve the overall efficacy of Contrave in managing weight.

**b. Behavioral Techniques:** An essential component of Contrave's strategy is behavioral counseling. In order to address issues including emotional eating, food cravings, and unhealthy eating behaviors, patients receive help on behavior change.

Behavioral techniques help people lose weight over time and give them the confidence to alter their lifestyles for the better.

**8. Particular Populations:**

**a. Senior Citizens:** The usage of Contrave in the elderly population is based on the patient's health status, co-occurring conditions, and the advantages and disadvantages of the medication.

When prescribing Contrave to older persons, factors such as altered metabolism and tolerance to medications are taken into account.

**b. Children's Population:** It is not recommended to use Contrave in pediatric patients. Its effectiveness and safety in those under a specific age, usually 18 years old, have not been shown.

Various factors need to be taken into account when devising weight management plans for children and teenagers. These may include nutritional counseling, lifestyle changes, and, in certain situations, prescription drugs that have been approved for use in children.

**9. Observation and Evaluations:**

**a. Frequent Observation:** People who are taking Contrave are routinely observed to evaluate their success in losing weight, their compliance with lifestyle changes, and the emergence of any adverse effects.
Weight, blood pressure, lipid profiles, and, in the case of diabetics, glycemic management are among the factors that may be monitored.

**b. Modifications to the Treatment:** Healthcare providers may modify the treatment strategy in response to continuing assessments. This could entail adjustments to the dosage of the medicine, adjustments to lifestyle advice, or, if necessary, consideration of stopping it altogether.

Contrave has been approved for use in treating adult obesity, managing comorbidities connected to weight, and lowering the risk of cardiovascular disease. The drug plays a more comprehensive function than just helping people lose weight; it incorporates behavioral methods and lifestyle improvements. Important components of guaranteeing the safe and efficient use of Contrave include patient selection criteria, educated decision-making, and continuous monitoring. Healthcare providers are essential in helping patients achieve sustainable weight management by helping them customize treatment programs, educating patients, and assisting them on their path, just like they would with any prescription drug.

# PATIENT ELIGIBILITY CRITERIA

The requirements for determining a patient's eligibility for Contrave, a medicine intended to aid in weight management, include a thorough evaluation of the patient's health status, medical history, and certain circumstances that may affect the medication's safety and effectiveness. In this comprehensive analysis, we examine the patient eligibility requirements for Contrave, taking into account elements including the degree of obesity, comorbidities, lifestyle factors, contraindications, and the significance of making well-informed decisions.

**1. BMI (body mass index) standards:**

**a. BMI Cutoff Points:** Body mass index (BMI), a statistic derived from a person's height and weight, is frequently used to assess a patient's eligibility for Contrave.
For those who are obese, defined as having a BMI of 30 kg/m² or more, contrave is usually taken into consideration. Furthermore, if a person has weight-

related comorbidities, they may be eligible if their BMI is equal to or higher than 27 kg/m².

**b. BMI and Severity of Obesity:** The degree of obesity, as measured by BMI, is a crucial factor in establishing a patient's eligibility. Greater potential benefits from Contrave in terms of weight management may be indicated by higher BMI values.

**2. Comorbidities Related to Weight:**

**a. Diabetes Mellitus Type 2:** People with type 2 diabetes mellitus who are obese may be able to use Contrave. Improvements in glycemic control and insulin sensitivity may follow from the medication's effects on weight control.

As part of the eligibility examination, medical professionals take diabetes severity and presence into account.

**b. dyslipidemia:** For obese people with dyslipidemia a condition marked by abnormal blood lipid levels Conveve may be an option.

The eligibility requirements for Contrave are influenced by improvements in lipid profiles linked to its usage, particularly for people with dyslipidemia.

**C. High blood pressure:** People who have high blood pressure and obesity might be able to use Contrave. Reductions in blood pressure resulting from weight loss with Contrave can help manage a common comorbidity of obesity.

When evaluating eligibility, criteria such as the degree of hypertension and its control are taken into account.

**3. Evaluation of Cardiovascular Risk:**

**a. Individual Risk Factors for Cardiovascular Disease:** A thorough evaluation of cardiovascular risk factors is essential for establishing a patient's eligibility. The purpose of prescribing Contrave may be to lower total cardiovascular risk.

Age, family history, smoking status, and pre-existing cardiovascular diseases are among the variables taken into account.

**b. Considering Cardiovascular Safety:** To determine whether using Contrave is safe, patients with pre-existing cardiovascular diseases or those who are more likely to experience cardiovascular events are carefully evaluated.

In the context of cardiovascular health, the possible advantages and disadvantages of weight control are evaluated.

**4. Factors related to lifestyle:**

**a. Dedication to Making Lifestyle Changes:** In order to be eligible for Contrave, a patient must make a commitment to changing their lifestyle, which may include eating differently, exercising more, and using behavioral techniques.
To optimize Contrave's efficacy, individuals must exhibit a willingness to actively participate in these lifestyle modifications.

**b. Behavior Therapy:** A fundamental component of Contrave's methodology is the integration of behavioral counseling. Behavioral treatments that target emotional eating, food cravings, and poor eating behaviors should be welcomed by eligible individuals.
Behavioral counseling improves Contrave's overall effectiveness in promoting long-term weight loss.

## 5. Smoking Patterns:

**a. A Look at Smoking Cessation:** Given that bupropion was initially prescribed as a smoking cessation aid, those who have smoked in the past or who smoke currently may be eligible for Contrave. One of the criteria for inclusion is the combined benefit of treating smoking cessation and weight management.

## 6. Restrictions:

**a. Complete Restrictions:** The use of Contrave may be completely prohibited by a few medical disorders or other considerations. For instance, because bupropion is linked to seizures, those with an active seizure disease or a history of seizures are usually ineligible for Contrave.

Those who have a history of allergy to the medication's active ingredients or particular components may also be contraindicated.

**b. Contraindications during lactation and pregnancy:** Pregnant women are generally encouraged to use effective contraception while taking the medicine, and contrave is not suggested at all during this time.

Additionally, because breastfeeding may allow the active elements in Contrave to pass to the baby, it is not advised during therapy.

**7. Renal and Hepatic Function:**

**a. The Hepatic Function:** Because Contrave is metabolized by the liver, hepatic function is taken into account when determining a patient's eligibility. It's possible that those with significant liver damage won't be able to use Contrave.
The evaluation of hepatic health and liver function tests inform the eligibility decision.

**b. Renal Function:** Although renal impairment is not a major problem when using Contrave, it may have an impact on dose modifications or the use of weight management techniques in some situations.

**8. A Look at Pediatric and Geriatric Issues:**

**a. Senior Citizens:** In the geriatric population, factors such as age-related changes in metabolism, medication tolerance, and general health status are taken into account when determining a patient's eligibility.

In older individuals, the possible advantages and disadvantages of using Contrave are carefully considered.

**b. Children's Population:** It is not recommended to use Contrave in pediatric patients. Its effectiveness and safety in those under a specific age, usually 18 years old, have not been shown.

Various factors need to be taken into account when devising weight management plans for children and teenagers. These may include nutritional counseling, lifestyle changes, and, in certain situations, prescription drugs that have been approved for use in children.

## 9. Patient Information and Well-Informed Choices:

**a. Consent that is informed:** In order for a patient to be eligible for Contrave, informed consent must be obtained. People should be given comprehensive information about the medicine, including its mode of action, any side effects, and the significance of changing one's lifestyle.

Patients are guaranteed active participation in the decision-making process through informed consent.

**b. Discussion of Risks and Benefits:** Healthcare providers have conversations regarding the possible advantages and disadvantages of Contrave with qualified patients. Patients are informed about the anticipated results of weight management initiatives, as well as any potential adverse effects and contraindications.

Encouraging people to make knowledgeable decisions regarding their health is the aim.

## 10. Observation and Succession:

**a. Continuous Evaluation:** Eligibility for a patient is determined continuously rather than all at once. The continuation or adjustment of Contrave treatment is guided by regular monitoring of weight loss progress, adherence to lifestyle modifications, and the development of side effects.

The treatment plan is modified in accordance with each patient's response and state of health.

**b. Considerations for Discontinuation:** If, after a given length of treatment, patients do not lose a predetermined quantity of weight, the option to stop taking Contrave is taken into consideration. Discontinuation may also be prompted by other circumstances, such as side effects or changes in health status.

The process of stopping something requires serious thought and could involve trying different approaches to managing weight.

Determining a patient's eligibility for Contrave necessitates a comprehensive evaluation of various aspects, including the degree of obesity, weight-related comorbidities, cardiovascular risk, lifestyle choices, contraindications, and specific health concerns. A customized assessment of each patient is used to determine whether to prescribe Contrave, with an emphasis on finding the best possible balance between the drug's possible advantages and disadvantages. The eligibility and treatment procedure for Contrave involves several crucial elements, including patient education, informed decision-making, and continued monitoring. Healthcare providers are essential in helping people go through this process and making sure Contrave is taken as part of a comprehensive weight-management plan in a safe and efficient manner.

# RECOMMENDED DOSAGE

A key component of the safe and efficient administration of the medicine Contrave, which is intended to help with weight management, is adhering to the appropriate dosage. The patient's response, tolerability, and particular circumstances pertaining to the medication's active ingredients bupropion and naltrexone are taken into account while determining the dosing schedule. In this thorough investigation, we examine the ideal Contrave dosage, taking into account start-up, titration, maintenance, particular populations, and prospective modifications based on clinical response.

**1. Starting a Treatment:**

**a. Initial Dosage:** When commencing a Contrave regimen, the starting dose is progressively increased until the desired maintenance dose is reached. In order to increase patient tolerance and reduce the possibility of side effects, the starting dose is usually smaller.

When establishing the initial dose, healthcare experts take into account individual considerations such as pre-existing medical conditions, comorbidities, and possible drug interactions.

**b. Slow Titration:** Over several weeks, Contrave is frequently titrated gradually to the desired maintenance dose. People can get used to the drug during this titration phase, which also lowers the possibility of adverse effects.

Healthcare practitioners can evaluate patient reaction and make necessary adjustments during the progressive titration.

**2. Goal Maintenance Level:**

**a. The Ideal Dose for Controlling Weight:** The ideal dosage at which Contrave is anticipated to have the greatest impact on weight control is known as the target maintenance dose. The data from clinical trials, evaluations of efficacy, and factors pertaining to the reaction of each patient individually are used to calculate this dose.

Patients are kept on the maintenance dose for the length of their treatment, which is often reached following the titration phase.

**b. Customized Method:** Contrave's suggested dosage considers the individualization principle. Patients may require different maintenance doses, and doctors will modify the dosage in response to many parameters, including clinical response overall, side effects, and the rate at which weight loss is occurring.

Every patient will receive the most efficient and well-tolerated dosage thanks to individualization.

### 3. Special Populations' Dosage Considerations:

**a. Senior Citizens:** The elderly population is subject to special considerations, and age-related factors may need adjusting the recommended dosage of Contrave. Changes in medication tolerance and metabolism are possible in older persons.

When choosing the right dosage for patients in the senior age range, healthcare providers carefully weigh the advantages and disadvantages.

**b. Children's Population:** It is not recommended to use Contrave in pediatric patients. It has not been determined whether the drug is safe or effective in people younger than a specific age, usually 18 years old.

Various factors need to be taken into account when devising weight management plans for children and teenagers. These may include nutritional counseling, lifestyle changes, and, in certain situations, prescription drugs that have been approved for use in children.

**4. Dosage Modification in Response to Clinical Response:**

**a. Progress in Losing Weight:** Continuous evaluations of the rate of weight reduction serve as a guide for changing the dosage of Contrave. Medical specialists assess the patient's degree of weight loss and determine whether the present dosage is having the desired effect.

Dosage changes may be taken into consideration to maximize the medication's effectiveness if weight loss is insufficient.

**b. Side effects and tolerability:** The occurrence of adverse effects and the patient's tolerance are important considerations when adjusting the dosage. If someone is having negative affects, the dosage may need to be changed, either by lowering the dose or by thinking about other options.

Frequent adverse effects of Contrave include headache, nausea, and constipation. Treatment success and patient adherence are enhanced by keeping an eye on and managing these side effects.

**5. Treatment Duration:**

**a. Extended-Term Administration:** Contrave isn't meant to be used temporarily; it's meant to be used for long-term weight management. Based on the patient's response to the drug, compliance with lifestyle changes, and continuous evaluation of benefits and hazards, the length of treatment is customized.

Decisions about whether to continue, modify, or stop using Contrave are guided by ongoing observation and reevaluation on a regular basis.

**b. Considerations for Discontinuation:** The amount of weight lost, side effects, and changes in the patient's health status are all taken into consideration while deciding whether to stop taking Contrave.

Medical practitioners determine if continued therapy is necessary, and in order to reduce the possibility of withdrawal symptoms, stopping a medicine may require a slow tapering off.

**6. Respect for Dosage Guidelines:**

**a. Patient Instruction:** Patient education makes it easier for patients to follow the dosage guidelines for Contrave. People are given comprehensive information regarding possible adverse effects, the careful titration procedure, and the significance of taking the drug as prescribed.

By encouraging a collaborative approach, patient education makes sure that patients are actively involved in their treatment plan.

**b. Counseling for Changes in Lifestyle:** In addition to dosage recommendations for Contrave, counseling on lifestyle modifications such as food adjustments and increased physical activity is recommended. Following through on these lifestyle adjustments improves Contrave's overall ability to help people lose weight.

In order to treat emotional eating and encourage healthy habits, behavioral measures are also highlighted.

## 7. Safety Surveillance:

**a. Frequent Observation:** A vital part of the Contrave treatment is routine monitoring. Medical personnel monitor vital signs like blood pressure and heart rate, analyze side effects, and evaluate the extent of weight loss.
By helping to identify possible problems early, safety monitoring makes it possible to intervene quickly and modify the treatment plan.

**b. Management of Adverse Events:** A component of safety monitoring is the handling of unfavorable incidents. In order to improve patient tolerance, healthcare providers swiftly address side effects and take supportive measures or dosage modifications into account.
For the purpose of reporting and handling adverse events, patient-provider communication is crucial.

## 8. Interaction with Additional Drugs:

**a. Considering Drug Interactions:** Potential medication interactions may have an impact on the recommended dosage for Contrave. Medical practitioners closely monitor the co-administration

of additional medications in order to prevent side effects or interactions that could impact drug metabolism.
Comprehensive treatment requires open communication with patients regarding all medications, including over-the-counter pharmaceuticals and vitamins.

The recommended dosage for Contrave is a meticulously planned regimen that takes into account individual considerations for initiation, titration, and maintenance. To get the best weight control results while maintaining patient safety and tolerability, the dosage is customized. Pediatric and elderly groups require special considerations, and dose modifications may be necessary in response to continuing evaluations of adherence and clinical response. The holistic approach to Contrave dose recommendations includes patient education, counseling on lifestyle modifications, safety monitoring, and knowledge of potential drug interactions. Healthcare experts are essential in helping patients through the treatment process with Contrave, just like they do with any prescription drug. They make sure that Contrave is administered safely and successfully within the framework of a comprehensive weight control plan.

## ADMINISTRATION GUIDELINES

The safe and efficient use of Contrave, a drug intended to help manage weight, is greatly dependent on following the administration instructions. These recommendations include a wide range of topics, such as missed dosage considerations, probable interactions, administration schedules, and whether or not to administer medication with food. In this in-depth investigation, we go into the detailed Contrave administration recommendations, providing information on how individuals and medical professionals can successfully integrate this medication into a patient's weight management regimen.

**1. Dosage Schedule:**

**a. One-Time Dosage Administration:** Usually, Contrave is used once a day. The drug regimen is made simpler by the once-daily dose schedule, which improves patient adherence.

The efficacy of Contrave in aiding with weight management is partly attributed to its regular administration at the same time every day.

**b. When to Take It:** Depending on personal preferences and lifestyle variables, there may be variations in the timing of Contrave administration. To minimize any potential changes to sleep patterns and to coincide with circadian cycles, it is normally advised to take Contrave at the same time every morning.

Specific advice may be given by medical specialists in light of each patient's circumstances and preferences.

**2. Delivery of Meals or Not:**

**a. Handling Food Administration:** It is possible to take Contrave with or without food. Food consumption may have an impact on the medicine's active ingredients, bupropion and naltrexone, although overall, the effect on medication efficacy is thought to be negligible.

When using Contrave, some people find that eating food helps reduce the unpleasant side effects of the medication, such as nausea and stomach pain.

**b. Uniform Guidelines for Administration:** Whether taking Contrave with or without food, people are recommended to maintain regular administration conditions for best outcomes. Predictable medication absorption and metabolism are supported by consistent administration circumstances.

**3. Procedure for Titration:**

**a. Slow Titration:** The Contrave dosage is titrated by gradually increasing it over a few weeks. This method lowers the possibility of adverse effects while allowing patients to adjust to the medicine.

Healthcare providers usually give the titration schedule, which details the precise dosage adjustments to be made at different intervals.

**b. Advice for Healthcare Professionals:** When it comes to helping patients through the titration process, healthcare professionals are essential. They make sure people comprehend and adhere to the suggested titration schedule by giving clear instructions on when to change the dosage.

During titration, routine follow-up visits enable medical professionals to monitor patient reaction and handle any issues or adverse effects.

## 4. Modifications in Dosage:

**a. Based on the Progress of Weight Loss:** Dosage changes might be taken into consideration depending on each person's rate of weight loss. Healthcare providers could consider modifying the Contrave dosage if the intended weight loss results are not realized.

Decisions about dosage adjustments are guided by ongoing assessments and regular monitoring of weight loss.

**b. Side effects and tolerability:** A crucial consideration in dosage modifications is patient tolerability. In the event that patients encounter adverse reactions, medical practitioners should think about lowering the dosage or looking into other options.

Frequent adverse effects of Contrave include headache, nausea, and constipation. Promoting patient adherence and the general success of treatment requires addressing these side effects.

## 5. Absence of Doses:

**a. The Value of Adherence:** The success of Contrave depends on following the recommended dose regimen. It is advised that patients take their medication on a regular basis and not miss any doses.

Missed doses may have an effect on treatment continuation and the accomplishment of weight management objectives.

**b. Regaining Missed Doses:** People are usually recommended to take the next planned dose of Contrave at the usual time if a dose is missed. It is not advised to take more medication or double the dosage in order to catch up.

Healthcare practitioners offer advice on how to handle missing doses, and patients should contact them as soon as they have any queries or concerns.

**6. Particular Populations:**

**a. Senior Citizens:** The elderly population is subject to special considerations, and age-related variables may need modifying the administration protocols. Changes in medication tolerance and metabolism are possible in older persons.

Healthcare practitioners carefully consider the advantages and disadvantages before deciding on the best administration guidelines for elderly patients.

**b. Children's Population:** It is not recommended to use Contrave in pediatric patients. It has not been determined whether the drug is safe or effective in people younger than a specific age, usually 18 years old.

Various factors need to be taken into account when devising weight management plans for children and teenagers. These may include nutritional counseling, lifestyle changes, and, in certain situations, prescription drugs that have been approved for use in children.

**7. Observation and Safety Measures:**

**a. Frequent Observation:** Throughout the Contrave therapy period, routine monitoring is crucial. Medical personnel monitor vital signs like blood pressure and heart rate, analyze side effects, and evaluate the extent of weight loss.

By helping to identify possible problems early, safety monitoring makes it possible to intervene quickly and modify the treatment plan.

**b. Management of Adverse Events:** A component of safety monitoring is the handling of unfavorable incidents. In order to improve patient tolerance, healthcare providers swiftly address side effects and take supportive measures or dosage modifications into account.

For the purpose of reporting and handling adverse events, patient-provider communication is crucial.

## 8. Interaction with Additional Drugs:

**a. Considering Drug Interactions:** Potential medication interactions may have an impact on Contrave's administration instructions. Medical practitioners closely monitor the co-administration of additional medications in order to prevent side effects or interactions that could impact drug metabolism.

Comprehensive treatment requires open communication with patients regarding all medications, including over-the-counter pharmaceuticals and vitamins.

## 9. Getting pregnant and nursing:

**a. Precautions for Pregnancy:** Pregnant women are generally encouraged to use effective contraception while taking the medicine, and contrave is not suggested at all during this time.

When someone becomes pregnant, whether it's unexpected or planned, they should get in touch with their healthcare professional right away to talk about possible treatment options and appropriate management.

**b. Considering Lactation:** Because breastfeeding could expose the newborn to the active ingredients in Contrave, it is not recommended during therapy. For breastfeeding moms, healthcare providers offer advice on alternate feeding options.

## 10. Considerations for Discontinuation:

**a. Tapering Off Gradually:** Healthcare providers could advise a slow tapering of Contrave rather than an abrupt stop if stopping the medicine is necessary. This strategy lessens the possibility of withdrawal symptoms.

The patient's health status changes, side effects, and amount of weight lost are all taken into account while making a decision about stopping treatment.

**b. Continuous Assistance:** In order to guarantee a seamless transition, stopping Contrave may require continuing help and supervision. Health care providers offer advice on how to keep up weight control techniques and handle any issues or problems that might surface after stopping.

The Contrave administration guidelines include a wide range of topics, including safety monitoring, missed doses, particular populations, and titration procedures and schedules for dosing. The purpose of these instructions is to help ensure that Contrave is used safely and effectively within the framework of an all-encompassing weight-management program. The success of Contrave treatment is largely attributed to the individualization of administration guidelines, routine monitoring, and open communication between patients and healthcare providers. Following administration instructions is crucial for maximizing results and fostering general patient well-being, just like it is with any prescription drug.

# EFFICACY STUDIES

The foundation for comprehending the efficacy of the medicine Contrave, which is intended for weight management, is provided by efficacy trials. In order to evaluate the effect of Contrave on weight loss, the amelioration of comorbidities associated with obesity, and overall patient outcomes, these studies entail thorough scientific inquiry. We examine the most important Contrave efficacy studies in-depth in this analysis, providing insight into the design, findings, and practical applications of the drug.

**1. Synopsis of Efficacious Research:**

**a. Trials with randomized controls (RCTs):** Randomized controlled trials (RCTs) are the cornerstone of Contrave efficacy investigations. Because RCTs are meant to reduce biases and confounding variables, they offer a reliable way to assess Contrave's efficacy in comparison to a control group.
These studies are usually carried out for predetermined amounts of time, with participant populations that have been carefully chosen and thorough result evaluations.

**b. Controlled Studies with Placebos:** Numerous Contrave efficacy studies use a placebo-controlled methodology. This enables researchers to compare Contrave's effects against a placebo in order to evaluate the drug's specific contribution. In order to assess the actual effects of Contrave, an inactive drug is given to the placebo group.

**c. Long-Term Research:** When evaluating if Contrave's effects are long-lasting, longitudinal studies are essential. Continuous monitoring and follow-up evaluations are part of these studies, which offer insights into changes in obesity-related comorbidities and the sustainability of weight loss.

**2. Efficient Loss of Weight:**

**a. Considerable Loss of Body Weight:** Studies on the effectiveness of Contrave regularly show that it significantly lowers body weight when compared to a placebo. A standardized way to quantify the effectiveness of a treatment is to express the amount of weight lost as a percentage of the starting body weight.

One important factor that influences Contrave's approval and uptake in clinical practice is how well it works for weight loss.

**b. Effects Dependent on Dose:** The effects of Contrave on weight loss in relation to dose are examined in several research. To find the ideal ratio between tolerance and efficacy, various dose regimens are compared.

When developing individualized treatment plans, healthcare providers can benefit greatly from the knowledge provided by dose-response correlations.

**3. Cardiometabolic Risk Factors Have Improved:**

**a. Effect on Profiles of Lipids:** The benefits of Contrave go beyond weight reduction to include changes in cardiometabolic risk factors. Research frequently evaluate the effect of the drug on lipid profiles, such as decreases in triglycerides, LDL cholesterol, and total cholesterol.

Positive alterations in lipid markers add to the overall decrease in cardiovascular risk that comes with using Contrave.

**b. Insulin sensitivity and glucose regulation:** Insulin sensitivity and glycemic control are frequently compromised in obese individuals. Studies on Contrave's effectiveness look at how it affects insulin sensitivity, glucose metabolism, and type 2 diabetes mellitus indicators.

Glycemic control improvements are especially important for obese people who also have other conditions like insulin resistance.

**4. Assessment of Comorbidities Associated with Obesity:**

**a. Effect on High Blood Pressure:** One prevalent comorbidity of obesity is hypertension. Studies examining Contrave's effectiveness measure drops in blood pressure, both diastolic and systolic.
For those who are obese and have high blood pressure, the possibility that Contrave will help regulate blood pressure is important.
**b. Impacts on Apnea of Sleep:** Sleep apnea is linked to a higher risk in obese people. A few efficacy studies examine how Contrave affects the symptoms and severity of sleep apnea.
Reductions in the severity of sleep apnea may have an impact on enhancing general wellbeing and sleep quality.

## 5. Quality of Life Affected by Health:

**a. Results as reported by patients:** Evaluations of health-related quality of life using patient-reported outcomes are frequently included in efficacy studies. These results demonstrate how Contrave affects people's ability to perform physically, emotionally, and in social situations, among other areas of their lives.

Enhancement of health-related quality of life is an important outcome that extends beyond measurements of physiological changes.

## 6. Twofold Mechanism of Action:

**a. The Function of Bupropion in Quitting Smoking:** One of Contrave's main chemicals, bupropion, was first created as a smoking cessation tool. Studies on the effectiveness of Contrave examine its combined benefits for managing weight and quitting smoking.

The evaluation of smoking cessation results gives Contrave's efficacy profile a special twist.

### 7. Analysis of Patient Subgroups:

**a. Subgroups by Gender, Age, and BMI:** Subgroup analyses in efficacy studies provide light on possible differences in Contrave's effects according to age, gender, and starting body mass index. The aforementioned analyses enhance our comprehension of Contrave's effectiveness in various patient demographics.

Healthcare providers can more effectively customize treatment recommendations by recognizing variations in response within subgroups.

### 8. Tolerance and Safety:

**a. Profile of Adverse Events:** A thorough evaluation of the safety and tolerability of Contrave is part of efficacy trials. The profiles of adverse events are meticulously recorded, emphasizing the identification of possible side effects.

The frequency and severity of common side effects, like nausea and constipation, are described.

**b. Assessments of Cardiovascular Safety:** Considering the link between cardiovascular risk and obesity drugs, effectiveness studies frequently

incorporate specific cardiovascular safety evaluations. Monitoring cardiac events, such as heart rate and rhythm, is part of these examinations.
A crucial component of Contrave's total risk-benefit analysis is its cardiovascular safety profile.

**9. Studies on Comparative Effectiveness:**

**a. Comparing This Weight Management Intervention with Others:** Certain efficacy studies provide Contrave's relative effectiveness by contrasting it with other weight-management strategies. These investigations could compare Contrave directly to other drugs or evaluate its efficacy when combined with lifestyle changes.
When evaluating treatment alternatives, healthcare practitioners can benefit greatly from the information provided by comparative effectiveness studies.

**10. After-Market Monitoring**

**a. Practical Efficiency and Security:** When evaluating the safety and efficacy of Contrave in the real world, post-marketing surveillance is essential. During this stage, the drug's usage in a larger population will be observed, outside of the carefully regulated setting of clinical trials.

Extended post-commercial monitoring offers valuable perspectives on Contrave's efficacy across a range of patient demographics and pinpoints any infrequent or enduring safety issues.

Research on the effectiveness of Contrave offers a thorough comprehension of its influence on weight reduction, amelioration of comorbidities associated with obesity, and general health outcomes for patients. Robust evidence is provided by longitudinal assessments, placebo-controlled trials, and randomized controlled trials to support the efficacy of Contrave in clinical practice. The assessment of health-related quality of life, obesity-related comorbidities, and cardiometabolic risk factors enhances the clinical picture and helps medical practitioners manage obese patients individually. Post-marketing surveillance keeps providing actual data, guaranteeing continuous observation of Contrave's efficacy and safety across a range of demographics. Contrave is positioned by the body of efficacy research as a useful tool in the multimodal approach to weight management, with potential benefits for enhancing the general well-being and physical health of those who struggle with obesity.

# SAFETY AND TOLERABILITY

Every medication, including the prescription drug Contrave, which is intended to help with weight management, must have both safety and tolerability. For those considering or currently using Contrave, as well as healthcare professionals, it is imperative to comprehend the medication's safety and tolerability profile. We examine many aspects of Contrave's safety and tolerability in this in-depth analysis, including adverse events, cardiovascular safety, possible hazards, contraindications, specific populations, and long-term usage considerations.

**1. Profile of Adverse Events:**

**a. Typical Adverse Reactions:** Like many other drugs, contrave may have typical adverse effects. These symptoms can include dry mouth, headache, nausea, constipation, and dizziness or sleeplessness. When evaluating the overall tolerance of Contrave, it is important to take into account the frequency and severity of these adverse effects.

**b. Handling Nausea:** One of the most common side effects of Contrave that people describe is nausea.

Taking Contrave with food, starting at a low dose during the initiation phase, and, if needed, exploring anti-nausea drugs are some techniques for managing nausea.

Healthcare practitioners offer direction on managing nausea in order to improve patient compliance and well-being.

**c. Impact on the Digestive System:** Another gastrointestinal adverse effect of Contrave is constipation. Encouragement of a healthy diet, plenty of water, and physical exercise can all help reduce constipation.

In order to manage gastrointestinal side effects and ensure appropriate interventions, it is imperative that healthcare providers and patients communicate effectively.

**d. Pain and Additional Neurological Repercussions:** Some Contrave users have reported experiencing headaches and dizziness. Usually, these neurological side effects are minor and temporary.

Throughout Contrave treatment, the general comfort and well-being of the patient is enhanced by the monitoring and management of headache and dizziness.

**e. Parched Mouth:** One typical adverse effect that people may have when using Contrave is dry mouth. Promoting proper oral hygiene and drinking plenty of water can help reduce the symptoms of dry mouth.

When determining how tolerable Contrave is, consideration is given to how dry mouth affects day-to-day activities and quality of life.

**2. Heart-related Safety:**

**a. Monitoring of Heart Rate and Blood Pressure:** A major area of emphasis for the Contrave review is cardiovascular safety. During clinical trials, routine blood pressure and heart rate monitoring is carried out, and this monitoring may continue throughout the course of treatment.

The effects of contrave on heart rate and blood pressure are thoroughly evaluated in order to identify any possible cardiovascular hazards.

**b. Effect on the QT Interval:** In particular, the effect of the drug on the QT interval a gauge of cardiac repolarization is taken into account when evaluating cardiovascular safety. Arrhythmias may be affected if the QT interval lengthens.

The continuous evaluation of Contrave's cardiovascular safety is aided by efficacy studies and post-marketing surveillance, especially in cases where the patient already has a cardiac problem.

**c. Those with cardiovascular conditions and safety:** For people with uncontrolled hypertension, a history of myocardial infarction, arrhythmias, or other serious cardiovascular disorders, contrave is usually not advised. Before writing a prescription for Contrave, medical practitioners thoroughly evaluate each patient's cardiovascular condition.

Cardiovascular safety also includes the monitoring of patients who already have cardiovascular disease while they are receiving therapy.

**3. Possible Dangers and Alerts:**

**a. Bupropion-Related Seizures:** One of the main chemicals of Contrave, bupropion, has been linked to a seizure risk. Those with a history of seizures or illnesses that reduce the threshold for seizures should be especially aware of this risk.

Seizures risk is assessed by medical professionals as part of Contrave contraindications and eligibility requirements.

**b. Suicidal Behaviors and Thoughts:** Antidepressant bupropion comes with a boxed warning about the elevated risk of suicide thoughts and actions. This caution applies to bupropion in all of its forms, including the one found in Contrave.

One of the most important aspects of patient safety throughout Contrave medication is keeping an eye out for any changes in behavior, mood, or suicidal thoughts.

**c. Possibility of both hyper- and hypoglycemia:** The effects of contrave on glucose metabolism are taken into account, and hypo- and hyperglycemia are possible outcomes. People with diabetes need to have their antidiabetic medication carefully monitored and adjusted as needed.

Healthcare professionals, endocrinologists, and primary care doctors must coordinate in order to manage Contrave collaboratively in persons with diabetes.

## 4. Restrictions:

**a. The past of seizures:** It is usually not recommended to use Contrave in people who have a history of seizures or who have medical problems that raise their risk of seizures.

The basis for the contraindication is the link between bupropion and a higher risk of seizures.

**b. Opioid Use Disorder and Eating Disorders:** In those with active eating disorders, contrave is contraindicated since it may worsen the psychological issues linked to these illnesses.

Because naltrexone in Contrave contains an opioid receptor antagonist, having an opioid use disorder is also contraindicated.

**c. Allergy and Hypersensitivity Reactions:** Contrave should not be used by anyone who has a history of known hypersensitivity to bupropion, naltrexone, or any of its ingredients.

Although they are uncommon, hypersensitivity reactions are regarded as contraindications.

**5. Particular Populations:**

**a. Senior Citizens:** Geriatric patients require special precautions, and using Contrave in older individuals requires a thorough evaluation of each patient's health status and tolerance to the drug.

Healthcare practitioners consider the possible advantages and disadvantages in light of aging-related changes in metabolism and general health.

**b. Children's Population:** It is not recommended to use Contrave in pediatric patients. It has not been determined whether the drug is safe or effective in people younger than a specific age, usually 18 years old.

Various factors need to be taken into account when devising weight management plans for children and teenagers. These may include nutritional counseling, lifestyle changes, and, in certain situations, prescription drugs that have been approved for use in children.

**6. Getting pregnant and nursing:**

**a. Precautions for Pregnancy:** Pregnant women are generally encouraged to use effective contraception while taking the medicine, and contrave is not suggested at all during this time.

When someone becomes pregnant, whether it's unexpected or planned, they should get in touch with their healthcare professional right away to talk about possible treatment options and appropriate management.

**b. Considerations for Breastfeeding:** Because breastfeeding could expose the newborn to the active ingredients in Contrave, it is not recommended during therapy. For breastfeeding moms, healthcare providers offer advice on alternate feeding options.

**7. Psychiatric Points to Remember:**

**a. Suicidal Behaviors and Thoughts:** Bupropion's boxed warning about a higher risk of suicide thoughts and actions highlights the importance of close observation, particularly in people with underlying mental health issues.
Throughout the Contrave therapy process, it is crucial for patients and mental health specialists to communicate closely.

**b. Possibility of Adverse Psychiatric Events:** Contrave may cause psychological side effects such as agitation, anxiety, and irritability. For prompt assistance and intervention, it's critical to keep an eye out for these occurrences, particularly during the beginning stage.

When mental health providers and medical specialists work together, it improves the overall care that people on Contrave receive.

## 8. Long-Term Use: Things to Think About

**a. Treatment Duration:** Contrave isn't meant to be used temporarily; it's meant to be used for long-term weight management. Based on the patient's response to the drug, compliance with lifestyle changes, and continuous evaluation of benefits and hazards, the length of treatment is customized.

Regular monitoring, safety evaluations, and consultations between patients and medical experts on treatment modifications or continuation are all part of long-term use considerations.

**b. Considerations for Discontinuation:** The amount of weight lost, side effects, and changes in the patient's health status are all taken into consideration while deciding whether to stop taking Contrave.

Medical practitioners determine if continued therapy is necessary, and in order to reduce the possibility of withdrawal symptoms, stopping a medicine may require a slow tapering off.

There are several factors to take into account while evaluating the safety and tolerability profile of Contrave, including potential hazards, adverse events, cardiovascular safety, particular populations, contraindications, and long-term usage considerations. When prescribing Contrave, medical providers must be aware of these factors, and patients must be educated when choosing a treatment strategy. A comprehensive weight control plan that includes ongoing monitoring, open communication, and collaborative management between patients and healthcare providers is crucial for the safe and effective use of Contrave. As with any drug, improving patient outcomes and fostering general well-being depend on ongoing assessments of safety and tolerability.

# COMMON ADVERSE REACTIONS

The safety and tolerability profile of Contrave, a medicine used for weight management, can be better understood by looking at common adverse responses linked to it. It's critical for medical experts as well as anyone thinking about using or considering the medicine to understand these typical adverse responses. We examine a number of frequent adverse reactions associated with Contrave in this in-depth analysis, including their prevalence, management approaches, and effects on patient adherence and treatment outcomes overall.

**1. Emesis:**

**a. Frequency and Incidence:** One of the most often reported side effects of Contrave is nausea. Both real-world data and clinical trials consistently show nausea as a common side effect.

Although it varies from person to person, nausea is usually more noticeable in the beginning stages.

**b. When and How Long It Takes:** Early on in the Contrave treatment regimen, particularly during the titration phase, nausea is frequently experienced. It usually subsides quickly, and many people report that their nausea decreases as they continue taking the drug.

**c. Techniques of Management:** Healthcare providers use a variety of techniques to treat Contrave-related nausea. These include suggesting that people take Contrave with food, lowering the starting dose, and, if required, thinking about using anti-nausea drugs.

Patient education about managing nausea improves adherence and assists people in coping with this frequent unpleasant event.

**2. Constipation:**

**a. occurrence:** Another commonly observed side effect linked to Contrave is constipation. It can cause discomfort and is typified by difficult or infrequent bowel movements.

Constipation varies in frequency among people, and tolerance is determined in part by how it affects day-to-day activities.

**b. Changes in Lifestyle:** Changes in lifestyle are frequently advised by medical specialists to relieve constipation. Increasing dietary fiber consumption, drinking plenty of water, and exercising frequently are a few examples.

Adherence to these lifestyle changes by patients helps to improve overall health and manage constipation.

## 3. Headache:

**a. Frequency and Intensity:** People who use Contrave frequently report experiencing headaches as an unpleasant response. Headaches can vary in frequency and intensity, but they are typically mild to moderate in severity.

Tracking the incidence and severity of headaches provide useful data for determining general tolerability.

**b. Passing Nature:** The headaches that come with using Contrave are frequently temporary and go away as people continue to take the drug. When assessing the overall effect on patient comfort, the length and pattern of headaches are taken into account.

**c. Use of Analgesics:** Under the advice of a healthcare provider, using over-the-counter analgesics for headache sufferers may be advised.

Effective headache management promotes patient adherence and satisfaction.

**4. Feeling lightheaded:**

**a. Rates and Set-Asides:** One typical side response with Contrave is reported to be dizziness. It could happen, especially when starting anything new or getting up rapidly.
Recognizing dizziness triggers, such as abrupt posture changes, helps medical providers offer specific management advice.
**b. Slow Adjustment:** Contrave-related dizziness is frequently transient, and most people get used to the drug over time. One way to manage this unfavorable reaction is to gradually change positions and increase fluid intake.

**5. Sleeplessness:**

**a. Sleep disturbances:** Sleep problems or insomnia have been reported as possible side effects of Contrave. People may have trouble going asleep, remaining asleep, or their sleep habits may alter.

The tolerability of Contrave is evaluated taking into account the effects of insomnia on day-to-day functioning and general well-being.

**b. When the Administration Will Act:** One tactic to reduce sleep problems is the timing of Contrave administration, especially avoiding taking the drug close to bedtime. Medical practitioners offer advice on how to best time dosages for people who are sleep deprived.

**6. Parched Mouth:**

**a. Impact and Frequency**: One of the most prevalent side effects of Contrave is dry mouth. It is typified by a feeling of parched mouth and could make things more uncomfortable.

When assessing the overall tolerance of dry mouth, factors such as its frequency and impact are taken into account.

**b. Drinking Suggestions:** To relieve dry mouth, recommendations for increasing fluid intake and practicing good oral hygiene are frequently made. These techniques aid in the management of this typical negative reaction.

## 7. Effect on Patient Compliance:

**a. Adverse Reaction Interaction:** Patient adherence depends on open communication about typical adverse responses between patients and healthcare providers. Realistic expectations are fostered by informing people about the anticipated side effects, their temporary nature, and possible control techniques.

**b. Obstacles to Adherence:** Adherence may face difficulties due to adverse reactions, even if they are frequent. In order to improve adherence, healthcare providers are essential in addressing issues, offering support, and modifying treatment regimens as necessary.

**c. Tailored Strategies:** Healthcare workers manage frequent adverse responses individually, understanding that people may have varied tolerance profiles. Depending on each patient's particular needs, changes in dose, lifestyle advice, or additional supporting measures may be taken into consideration.

**8. Effect on Life Quality:**

**a. Results as reported by patients:** Even though they are common, Contrave adverse effects might affect a person's quality of life in terms of their health. Patient-reported outcomes document the influence on different facets of people's lives, such as social relationships, emotional stability, and physical comfort.

A comprehensive understanding of the medication's overall tolerability benefits from tracking and resolving the influence on quality of life.

**b. Cooperative Decision-Making:** In shared decision-making, patients and medical professionals assess the possible advantages of Contrave for managing weight against the possible negative effects on quality of life. Treatment programs are guaranteed to be in line with each patient's preferences and goals thanks to this cooperative approach.

**9. Durability of Adverse Events:**

**a. Duration of Adverse Reactions:** Managing expectations requires an understanding of the duration of typical unfavorable reactions. As they continue using Contrave, many people report that the frequency and severity of their adverse effects decrease.

When unfavorable responses persist, medical practitioners know when to reevaluate and take treatment plan modifications into consideration.

**b. Evaluation and Adjustment:** Healthcare providers are guided in their decision-making on treatment plan modifications, dose adjustments, and further interventions through the periodic reevaluation of adverse events. The optimization of treatment outcomes and continued patient care are facilitated by this dynamic process.

**10. Interaction and Assistance:**

**a. Patient Instruction:** The key to controlling common adverse effects is patient education. Giving patients clear and thorough information about possible side effects, how they should progress, and proactive management techniques gives them more control over their medical journey.

**b. Assistive Interventions:** One of the most important things that healthcare professionals do is support patients and answer any worries they may have about bad responses. Collaboration, prompt communication, and attention to each patient's requirements all play a part in making the patient experience pleasant and encouraging.

A thorough picture of Contrave's safety and tolerability profile can be gained from common side events, which include nausea, constipation, headaches, dizziness, sleeplessness, and dry mouth. Despite their prevalence, these adverse responses are frequently temporary, and there are efficient management techniques available to improve patient comfort. Adverse responses have a significant impact on patient adherence, quality of life, and general well-being, which emphasizes the significance of tailored strategies and continuous communication between patients and medical staff. Healthcare providers enhance the overall treatment experience and assist patients in managing their weight with Contrave by anticipating and working together to address typical side events.

# SERIOUS SIDE EFFECTS

The prescription drug Contrave, which is intended to help with weight management, has serious adverse effects that need to be thoroughly investigated in order to fully grasp the risks involved. Medical practitioners, patients, and anybody considering or using the medicine must recognize and handle major side effects, even though they are less often than mild or temporary reactions. We examine a number of major side effects associated with Contrave in this comprehensive analysis, including their frequency, clinical consequences, risk factors, monitoring techniques, and implications for patients and healthcare providers.

**1. Convulsions:**

**a. Risk and Incidence Factors:** Given that bupropion is one of Contrave's active ingredients, seizures are acknowledged as a major adverse effect of the medication. Seizures are uncommon in general but become more common as bupropion dosages are increased.

Seizures have been linked to eating problems, excessive alcohol use, a history of seizures, and the use of drugs that decrease the threshold for seizures.

**b. Agents that Lower the Seizure Threshold:** Contrave increases the risk of seizures because some drugs, substances, or situations can lower the seizure threshold. Medical practitioners evaluate the possible interactions and modify treatment regimens as necessary.

**c. Clinical Consequences:** From possible harm during the seizure episode to the requirement for medical intervention, seizures can have major therapeutic ramifications. One of the most important aspects of patient safety when using Contrave is monitoring for seizures.

**d. Strategies for Monitoring:** Throughout the first assessment and the duration of Contrave medication, medical personnel keep an eye out for seizure risk in patients. It could be essential to work closely with neurologists or other specialists, particularly in cases where there has been a history of seizures.

**e. Modification of Dosage and Cessation:** When seizures happen, medical practitioners might think about changing the dosage or stopping the use of Contrave. Based on the entire risk-benefit analysis and the necessity of giving patient safety top priority, customized judgments are made.

**2. Suicidal Behaviors and Thoughts:**

**a. Cautionary Note in a Box:** One of Contrave's ingredients, bupropion, has a boxed warning on it about the elevated risk of suicidal thoughts and actions. This caution emphasizes the need for close observation and applies to all bupropion formulations.

**b. Mental Health Conditions:** Suicidal thoughts are one of the psychiatric adverse effects of Contrave that may be more likely to affect people who already have mental health issues. When providing treatment, medical experts evaluate the patient's past mental health history and keep a careful eye out for any changes.

**c. Watching for Shifts in Mood:** An essential component of the Contrave therapy protocol is monitoring for changes in mood, behavior, and suicidal thoughts. Prompt action and assistance are ensured by regular communication between healthcare professionals and individuals.

**d. Teamwork in Management:** For those with a history of mental health issues, collaborative management with mental health specialists can be required. Comprehensive patient care is facilitated by interdisciplinary teams and shared decision-making.

**3. Events Related to the Heart:**

**a. Heart rate and blood pressure:** Cardiovascular events, such as variations in heart rate and blood pressure, are taken into account when assessing Contrave's safety profile. It is important to keep an eye on these indicators, particularly in people who already have cardiovascular disease.

**b. QT Interval Extender:** One possible cardiac side effect of Contrave is prolongation of the QT interval, which is primarily related to bupropion. In people with cardiovascular risk factors, this impact should be carefully considered as it may raise the risk of arrhythmias.

**c. Entire Cardiovascular Evaluation:** Healthcare providers perform a thorough cardiovascular assessment before starting Contrave, taking into account the patient's medical history, present cardiovascular condition, and risk factors. Continuous cardiovascular safety is ensured by routine monitoring during treatment.

**d. Precautions for Heart Conditions:** In general, people with uncontrolled hypertension, a history of myocardial infarction, arrhythmias, or other serious cardiovascular disorders should not use contrave. People who are at risk of cardiovascular disease are protected with extra care.

**4. High blood pressure:**

**a. Frequency and Tracking**: One major possible side effect of Contrave is hypertension. Although everyone will experience it differently, blood pressure monitoring is crucial, particularly in the early stages and in people who already have hypertension.

**b. Customized Blood Pressure Objectives:** Specific blood pressure goals are set for each person according to their cardiovascular risk and current state of health. Healthcare practitioners take into account striking a balance between sustaining cardiovascular health and reaching weight control goals.

**c. Controlling High Blood Pressure:** Healthcare providers may change a patient's lifestyle, change the dosage of Contrave, or think about taking other antihypertensive drugs if hypertension develops.

Tailored strategies are essential for the best possible blood pressure control.

**5. Negative Impacts on Behavior and Mood:**

**a. Anxiety, irritability, and agitation:** The usage of contrave has been linked to negative consequences on behavior and mood, such as agitation, irritation, and worry. It's critical to keep an eye out for these side effects, particularly in the early stages of treatment.

**b. Mental Health Consultation:** Consulting a psychiatrist may be beneficial for individuals who are exhibiting notable changes in their mood and behavior. Healthcare providers collaborate to manage side effects, think about changing dosages, or investigate different approaches to treatment.

**c. Things to Think About for Psychiatric Conditions:** People with pre-existing psychiatric problems are subject to special considerations. The possible effects of Contrave on behavior and mood are carefully evaluated, and treatment regimens are modified with the patient's general mental health in mind.

**6. Possibility of both hyper- and hypoglycemia:**

**a. Effects of Glucose Metabolism:** There is a chance that contrave will affect glucose metabolism, possibly resulting in hyperglycemia or hypoglycemia. People with diabetes need to be closely watched, and their anti-diabetic medication may need to be changed.

**b. Cooperative Diabetes Care:** For diabetics using Contrave, collaborative care with endocrinologists or diabetes experts is crucial. Healthcare providers must work together to manage weight and glucose levels while focusing on both issues at the same time.

**c. Instruction for Patients on Blood Pressure Monitoring:** Patients taking Contrave for diabetes must get patient education on blood glucose self-monitoring. Being aware of possible variations in blood sugar allows people to take an active role in managing their diabetes.

**7. Hypersensitivity and Allergy Reactions:**

**a. Uncommon but Dangerous Reactions:** Despite being uncommon, allergic reactions and hypersensitivity to Contrave are regarded as significant conditions that might cause breathing difficulties, edema, or skin rashes. Medical treatment must be given to these responses right away.

**b. Safety Measures and Patient Instruction:** One way to reduce the possibility of allergic reactions is to thoroughly evaluate each patient's allergies before recommending Contrave. Timely intervention is encouraged by educating patients on how to recognize the indicators of allergic reactions.

**c. Stopping in the Event of Allergic Reactions:** It is essential to stop taking Contrave if allergic reactions or hypersensitivity occur. Medical professionals help people through the process and could look into different approaches to managing their weight.

## 8. A Rare yet Serious Adverse Event for the Liver

**a. Hepatotoxicity**: Hepatotoxicity, defined as adverse events connected to the liver, is regarded as an uncommon but potentially dangerous side effect of Contrave. These events might include increased liver enzyme levels and, in severe situations, liver failure.

**b. Tracking Liver Activity:** While taking Contrave, it is customary to monitor liver function. Frequent evaluations of liver enzymes aid in the early detection of hepatotoxicity and enable prompt intervention.

**c. Symptoms and Clinical Indications:** Health care providers inform patients about the warning signs and symptoms of adverse events connected to the liver, such as jaundice, abdominal discomfort, or unexplained lethargy. Early reporting of these symptoms enables timely diagnosis and treatment.

**9. Unfavorable Respiratory Events:**

**a. Uncommon Respiratory Issues:** When using Contrave, rare but serious respiratory side effects have been observed, such as dyspnea (difficulty breathing) and pneumonitis, which may need medical attention and medication withdrawal.

**b. Tracheal Monitoring:** Early detection is crucial to reducing potential problems, and individuals using Contrave are closely observed for respiratory symptoms, and medical professionals perform comprehensive exams if respiratory adverse events are anticipated.

**c. Things to Take Into Account for People with Respiratory Conditions:** Individuals who already have a respiratory problem are subject to special considerations. The possible effects of Contrave on respiratory function are carefully evaluated, and treatment plans are modified as necessary to guarantee patient safety.

**10. Unwanted Reactions in the Digestive System:**

**a. Effects of Naltrexone:** Naltrexone is a contributing component in the gastrointestinal side events associated with Contrave, which include nausea and constipation. Although these symptoms are often modest, it is important to monitor for more serious gastrointestinal issues.

**b. Communication Regarding Severe GI Symptoms:** People are informed about the possibility of experiencing severe gastrointestinal symptoms, like continuous stomach pain or vomiting, which could signal more serious issues. Effective communication encourages prompt medical intervention.

There are a number of serious side effects linked to Contrave that need to be carefully considered and monitored. These include seizures, suicidal thoughts and behaviors, cardiovascular events, hypertension, negative mood and behavior effects, the potential for hypo- and hyperglycemia, allergic reactions and hypersensitivity, hepatotoxicity, respiratory adverse events, and gastrointestinal adverse events. Healthcare professionals are essential in identifying individual risk factors, putting monitoring strategies into place, and promptly addressing serious side effects to ensure patient safety. Informed and customized treatment plans are also a result of shared decision-making, patient education, and a collaborative approach between individuals and healthcare professionals.

# CONDITIONS WHERE CONTRAVE IS NOT RECOMMENDED

Due to potential risks and contraindications, Contrave, a prescription medication intended for weight management, is not recommended in certain medical conditions. It is important for healthcare professionals to be aware of these conditions when prescribing Contrave, as well as for individuals who may be considering or using the medication. In this thorough analysis, we explore the conditions in which Contrave is not recommended, offering insights into the reasoning behind these recommendations, potential risks, and alternative weight management strategies.

**1. The Seizures' Past:**

**a. Justification:** Bupropion, an antidepressant and smoking cessation aid found in Contrave, has been linked to an increased risk of seizures. People who have previously experienced seizures are more likely to experience seizures when using Contrave.

The goal of the contraindication in those with a seizure history is to reduce the risk of complications from seizures.

**b. Evaluation of Seizure Risk:** During the initial evaluation, medical experts carefully evaluate each patient's risk of seizures. Determining contraindications requires a comprehensive medical history that includes any history of seizures or disorders that reduce the seizure threshold.

**d. Different Strategies:** Alternative approaches to weight management that do not use drugs associated with seizure risks may be taken into consideration for individuals with a history of seizures. Important elements of the treatment strategy include nutritional counseling, lifestyle adjustments, and other non-pharmacological treatments.

**2. Disorders Related to Eating:**

**a. Justification:** People who suffer from active eating disorders, such as bulimia nervosa and anorexia nervosa, may be more susceptible to psychological side effects when taking Contrave. Because of the medication's potential to affect mood and behavior, care should be used when administering this medication to this population.

The contraindication stems from the need to prevent aggravating mental health issues linked to eating disorders.

**b. Evaluation of the Psyche:** Healthcare providers identify patients with current eating disorders before writing a prescription for Contrave. This process helps to guide treatment options and protects patients who have particular psychological vulnerabilities.

**c. Interventions using Behavior:** As alternate weight-management treatments, behavioral therapies, psychotherapy, and nutritional counseling may be suggested for individuals with eating disorders. These approaches center on addressing the psychological issues that underlie disordered eating.

**3. Disorder of Opioid Use:**

**a. Justification:** Opioid receptor antagonists, such as naltrexone, which is a part of Contrave, have the potential to exacerbate withdrawal symptoms in people with opioid use disorders.

The purpose of the contraindication for people with opioid use disorders is to shield them from the negative consequences of opioid withdrawal.

**b. Risk of Opioid Withdrawal:** Getting a complete history of opioid use helps medical experts determine the likelihood of opioid withdrawal. People who have recently or now have an opioid use disorder are not recommended to use Contrave because of the danger of withdrawal symptoms.
Treatment for Substance Use Disorders:

Treatment methods for substance use disorders, such as medication-assisted treatment (MAT), counseling, and support groups, may be helpful to those with opioid use disorder. Contrave, because it contains an opioid receptor antagonist, is not advised for this population.

**4. Intolerance to Naltrexone or Bupropion:**

**a. Justification:** Allergy reactions can occur in people who have a known hypersensitivity to bupropion, naltrexone, or any of the ingredients in Contrave. Hypersensitivity reactions are uncommon but can be dangerous and can cause swelling, skin rashes, or breathing difficulties.
The contraindication serves as a safety precaution to reduce the possibility of hypersensitive responses.

**b. Allergy Evaluation:** Before writing a prescription for Contrave, medical practitioners check patients for known allergies to bupropion, naltrexone, or similar substances. Thorough allergy testing ensures that the drug is used safely.

**c. Complementary Medicines:** If a person has a hypersensitivity to any of the ingredients in Contrave, they may consider non-pharmacological methods or other weight-management medications. The choice of non-pharmacological methods will depend on the patient's health and treatment objectives.

## 5. Unmanaged High Blood Pressure:

**a. Justification:** Blood pressure may rise as a result of using Contrave. People who have uncontrolled hypertension are more likely to experience cardiovascular issues, and using Contrave in this population may make pre-existing conditions worse.

The purpose of the contraindication in uncontrolled hypertension is to protect people with high blood pressure.

**b. Tracking Blood Pressure:** Before starting Contrave, medical experts take a complete blood pressure reading. People with uncontrolled hypertension can benefit from blood pressure management measures before thinking about taking weight management drugs.

**c. Modifications to Lifestyle:** For those with uncontrolled hypertension, lifestyle treatments such as dietary adjustments, increased physical activity, and stress reduction are advised. These interventions improve cardiovascular health in general and may be given priority over the use of medication.

## 6. Background of Myocardial Ischemia and Additional Cardiovascular Disorders:

**a. Justification:** Cardiovascular events are more likely to occur in those with a history of myocardial infarction or other major cardiovascular diseases. Contrave may enhance the risk of cardiovascular events in this population due to its potential effects on blood pressure and heart rate.

The rationale behind the contraindication is the necessity of giving cardiovascular safety top priority in people with a history of cardiac incidents.

**b. Assessment of the Heart:** Healthcare providers perform a thorough cardiovascular assessment, which includes an examination of the patient's cardiovascular history, current cardiovascular condition, and risk factors, before writing a prescription for Contrave.

**c. Customized Risk Management for Cardiovascular Disease:** Individualized cardiovascular risk management becomes crucial for people with a history of myocardial infarction or cardiovascular diseases. Medical professionals work in conjunction with cardiologists or cardiovascular experts to optimize treatment regimens.

## 7. Application of MAOIs, or monoamine oxidase inhibitors:

**a. Justification:** Monoamine oxidase inhibitors (MAOIs) and Contrave both affect neurotransmitter levels, and using them together increases the risk of serious side effects. Therefore, using Contrave and MAOIs together increases the chance of interactions that could result in hypertensive crises.

The purpose of the contraindication is to shield MAOI users from potentially dangerous interactions.

**b. Review of Medication:** Healthcare providers examine patients' medical histories to determine whether they have used MAOIs. If they have, or have recently taken, MAOIs, Contrave is not started until the proper washout period has passed.

**c. Additional Antidepressant Choices:** Those in need of antidepressant therapy may want to look into safer alternatives to Contrave, such as selective serotonin reuptake inhibitors (SSRIs) or other antidepressants, depending on their specific needs and tolerance.

**8. Age**

**a. Justification:** Contrave is not recommended for use in children. The safety and effectiveness of the drug have not been proven in people under a specific age, usually 18 years old.

The age limit is based on the scant data that is currently available on Contrave use in pediatric populations.

**b. Techniques for Pediatric Weight Management:** Paediatric weight management is a multidisciplinary field that combines behavioral interventions, physical activity promotion, and dietary counseling. Physicians, dietitians, and other specialists work together to address weight-related issues in children and young adults.

## 9. Breastfeeding with Pregnancy:

**a. Justification:** There is insufficient information available on the possible dangers to the developing fetus or nursing infant, and the safety of Contrave during pregnancy and breastfeeding has not been established.

The contraindication is a safety safeguard to protect the unborn child or nursing baby from possible harm.

**b. Counseling on Contraception:** Health care providers counsel people who may become pregnant about contraception. Women who are considering getting pregnant are recommended to utilize an effective form of contraception while using Contrave.

**c. Considerations for Breastfeeding:** Healthcare professionals explore alternate weight control measures for nursing individuals in order to ensure the health and well-being of both the mother and the infant. Contrave is generally not recommended while breastfeeding.

## 10. Damage to the Renals:

**a. Justification:** Since both bupropion and naltrexone are metabolized in the liver and their pharmacokinetics may be changed in patients with renal failure, there has not been enough research done on the safety and effectiveness of Contrave in patients with end-stage renal disease or severe renal impairment.

The requirement for caution in people with compromised renal function forms the basis of the contraindication in severe renal impairment.

**b. Renal Function Evaluation:** Before administering Contrave, medical experts evaluate renal function. If a patient has renal impairment, other weight-management techniques or Contrave dosage changes may be taken into consideration.

**c. Working along with nephrologists:** When managing patients with renal impairment, multidisciplinary treatment ensures a complete approach to weight management while taking renal health into consideration. Collaboration with nephrologists or renal specialists is useful in this regard.

# DRUG INTERACTIONS

It is important for medical practitioners to understand drug interactions while administering Contrave, as well as for patients who may be considering or already using the medicine. The combination of bupropion and naltrexone known as Contrave may interact with other drugs, perhaps compromising their safety or effectiveness. We examine Contrave medication interactions in-depth in this investigation, offering information on mechanisms, clinical ramifications, monitoring techniques, and things to think about for both individuals and healthcare providers.

**1. Interactions between Cytochrome P450 (CYP) Enzymes:**

**a. The metabolism of bupropion:** The main metabolite of bupropion, an ingredient in Contrave, is cytochrome P450 2B6 (CYP2B6). Bupropion plasma concentrations can be influenced by drugs that either activate or inhibit CYP2B6.

Inducers like rifampin have the ability to lower bupropion levels, which could diminish its effectiveness. On the other hand, bupropion levels may rise in response to inhibitors like fluoxetine, requiring dose modifications.

**b. Metabolism of Naltrexone:** Hepatic enzymes are involved in the metabolism of naltrexone, with cytochrome P450 having a minor function. Drugs that impact hepatic function must be taken into account, even if CYP interactions are less relevant for naltrexone.

**c. Clinical Consequences:** When prescribing Contrave, medical practitioners consider interactions between CYP enzymes. It's critical to keep an eye out for any changes in effectiveness or adverse effects, and depending on the co-administered medications, dose modifications can be required.

**2. MAOIs, or monoamine oxidase inhibitors:**

**a. Hypertensive Crisis Risk:** Because of the possibility of hypertensive crises, using Contrave and MAOIs together is not recommended. Neurotransmitter levels are influenced by both bupropion and naltrexone, and their combination can have serious side effects.

The contraindication highlights how crucial it is to steer clear of dangerous interactions that could lead to potentially fatal complications.

**b. Review of Medication:** To determine whether MAOIs are being used, medical practitioners perform extensive medication reviews. When someone has recently taken or is now taking MAOIs, starting Contrave is postponed until the proper washout period has passed.

**c. Other Options for Antidepressants:** When combined with Contrave, non-risky alternatives can be investigated by those in need of antidepressant treatment. Depending on the demands of the patient and their tolerance, selective serotonin reuptake inhibitors (SSRIs) or other antidepressants may be recommended.

**3. Opioid Antagonists and Analgesics:**

**a. How Naltrexone Works:** Opioid receptor antagonists like Naltrexone, which is an ingredient in Contrave, can counteract the analgesic benefits of opioid drugs. Reduced pain alleviation from opioid receptor blockage may have an effect on how pain disorders are managed.

When using Contrave, people who are on long-term opioid medication or who need to handle acute pain should exercise caution.

**b. Risk of Opioid Withdrawal:** Because of the antagonistic effect of naltrexone, people who use opioid analgesics may have withdrawal symptoms while starting to use Contrave. Before beginning Contrave, opioids may need to be tapered off gradually or stopped entirely.

**c. Techniques for Pain Management:** Patients on Contrave and in need of opioid analgesics may benefit greatly from collaborative pain management including pain experts. It may be wise to explore different approaches to pain treatment or make modifications to opioid dosage plans.

**4. Psychotropic and antidepressant medications:**

**a. Risk of Serotonin Syndrome:** The risk of serotonin syndrome may increase if Contrave is taken with other drugs that raise serotonin levels. The signs of this potentially fatal illness include agitation, hallucinations, fast heartbeat, and heat exhaustion.

When providing Contrave along with other serotonergic drugs, medical practitioners evaluate the patient's risk for serotonin syndrome.

**b. Review of Medication:** A comprehensive evaluation of a patient's pharmaceutical regimen involves determining whether antidepressants, selective serotonin reuptake inhibitors (SSRIs), serotonin-norepinephrine reuptake inhibitors (SNRIs), and other psychotropic drugs are being used concurrently. It could be essential to make changes or stop altogether to avoid serotonin syndrome.

**c. Keeping an eye out for serotonin syndrome:** Serotonergic drug users on Contrave are kept an eye out for symptoms of serotonin syndrome. Reduced symptom severity and patient safety are dependent on early detection and treatments.

**5. Drugs that are antipsychotics:**

**a. Effects of Dopamine:** One of Contrave's ingredients, bupropion, has dopaminergic properties. When Contrave is taken alongside antipsychotic drugs, particularly those that block dopamine receptors, it may disrupt neurotransmitter balance and have an adverse effect on mental stability.

Medical practitioners evaluate the possibility of interactions and keep a careful eye on patients' psychiatric symptom changes.

**b. Psychiatric Evaluation:** One aspect of comprehensive mental health evaluations is determining whether or not a patient is using antipsychotic drugs. To maximize treatment regimens and handle any conflicts, collaborative management with psychiatrists can be required.

**c. Tailored Psychotropic Techniques:** Individualized psychotropic tactics are taken into consideration when interactions are an issue. Depending on the needs of the patient, antipsychotic drug adjustments, dose titrations, or other treatment approaches may be investigated.

**6. Antiplatelet agents and anticoagulants:**

**a. Risk of Bleeding:** One ingredient in Contrave, bupropion, may make bleeding more likely. Contrave may increase this risk when combined with anticoagulants or antiplatelet medicines, thus cautious monitoring is required.

When treating patients who need anticoagulant or antiplatelet medicine, healthcare providers evaluate the patient's bleeding risk and take alternate weight-management techniques into account.

**b. Monitoring Coagulation:** People using anticoagulant or antiplatelet drugs along with Contrave are watched for bleeding symptoms. Effective bleeding risk management involves working with haematologists and performing routine coagulation assessments.

**c. Customized Cardiovascular Risk Reduction:** Cardiologists or other cardiovascular experts can provide valuable collaborative management for patients who need anticoagulant or antiplatelet therapy in addition to Contrave. Thorough cardiovascular risk management is ensured via interdisciplinary treatment.

**7. Medicines for Antidiabetes:**

**a. Effects of Glucose Metabolism:** The effects of Contrave on the metabolism of glucose may interfere with anti-diabetic drugs. In those with diabetes, there is a risk of hypo- or hyperglycemia, thus close monitoring is necessary.

When starting Contrave, medical experts evaluate the patient's diabetic management plan and work in tandem with endocrinologists.

**b. Glycemic Management Tracking:** When taking Contrave, diabetics have their glycemic control closely monitored. To optimize glucose levels, changes may be required to insulin regimes, anti-diabetic medicines, or lifestyle choices.

**c. Cooperative Decision-Making:** A shared decision-making process between patients, medical providers, and endocrinologists guarantees that glycemic control tactics and weight management objectives are in sync. Treatment modifications based on each patient's response are guided by open communication.

**8. Medication for hypertension:**

**a. Effects of Blood Pressure:** It is possible for Contrave to raise blood pressure. Blood pressure regulation may be impacted by taking Contrave along with antihypertensive drugs, necessitating modifications to antihypertensive regimens.
In order to optimize hypertension management, healthcare workers measure blood pressure measurements and work in conjunction with specialists or primary care physicians.
**b. Customized Blood Pressure Objectives:** Setting specific blood pressure goals becomes essential for people using antihypertensive drugs in addition to Contrave. Discussions about treatment objectives and modifications depending on total cardiovascular risk are part of shared decision-making.

**c. Changes in Lifestyle:** It is advised that people on Contrave and antihypertensive drugs alter their lifestyles to include eating healthier, exercising more, and reducing stress. All things considered, these therapies improve cardiovascular health.

**9. Hormonal Birth Control:**

**a. Possible Correspondences:** One ingredient in Contrave, bupropion, may interact with hormonal contraceptives, influencing how they are metabolized. It is necessary to take into account the possibility of reduced contraceptive efficacy in people who use both drugs.
In order to achieve successful birth control while using Contrave, healthcare providers work with gynecologists and discuss contraceptive options.

**b. Counseling on Contraception:** When starting Contrave, those who are potentially fertile are given contraception advice. Depending on personal preferences and requirements, other methods of contraception or modifications to hormonal contraceptive regimens may be taken into consideration.

**c. Checking the Effectiveness of Contraceptives:** For those using both hormonal and Contrave contraceptives, continuous monitoring of the effectiveness of the contraceptive method is crucial. Individual responses may dictate the need for modifications to contraceptive methods or the addition of additional measures.

**10. Lipid-Lowering Drugs and Statins:**

**a. Effects of Lipid Profile:** Contrave may have an impact on cholesterol levels and lipid profiles. It is necessary to keep an eye out for changes in lipid parameters when taking Contrave in combination with statins or other lipid-lowering drugs.
To maximize cholesterol management, healthcare practitioners evaluate lipid profiles and work with lipid specialists.
**b. Customized Lipid Objectives:** For those using cholesterol-lowering drugs such as Contrave, setting personalized lipid targets is crucial. Discussions about treatment objectives and modifications depending on total cardiovascular risk are part of shared decision-making.
**c. Changes in Lifestyle:** For those using lipid-lowering drugs such as Contrave, lifestyle adjustments such as dietary adjustments, greater physical activity, and quitting smoking are advised.

All things considered, these therapies improve cardiovascular health.

It is critical for both individuals and healthcare professionals to comprehend drug interactions pertaining to Contrave. The complexity of pharmacological interactions is highlighted by the interactions that are discussed, which include those involving CYP enzymes, monoamine oxidase inhibitors (MAOIs), opioid analgesics, antipsychotic and antidepressant drugs, anticoagulants and antiplatelet agents, antidiabetic drugs, hormonal contraceptives, statins, and lipid-lowering drugs. In order to achieve safe and efficient weight management with Contrave, healthcare professionals are essential in performing comprehensive medication reviews, evaluating individual risk factors, and putting monitoring systems into place. Health care providers and patients can create individualized treatment programs that put the patient's overall health and weight control objectives first by collaborating on decisions and communicating openly.

# SPECIAL CONSIDERATIONS

There are subtle factors related to the use of Contrave that people should be aware of when thinking about or using the medicine, and healthcare practitioners must be aware of while prescribing it. These elements include a wide range of things, such as age- and gender-specific characteristics, cultural factors, comorbid conditions, and particular demographics, including pregnant people. In this thorough investigation, we dive into the unique aspects related to Contrave, providing insights into the complex nature of these elements and their significance for individuals as well as healthcare professionals.

**1. Age-Specific Things to Consider:**

**a. Adolescent and Pediatric Populations:** It is generally not recommended to use Contrave in pediatric patients. There is little information available about its effectiveness and safety in those under a specific age, usually 18 years old.

A multidisciplinary strategy that incorporates behavioral interventions, physical activity promotion, and nutritional counseling is used to manage weight in children.

**b. Considering the Elderly:** Age-related changes in metabolism, renal function, and other physiological processes can occur in older persons. When prescribing Contrave to elderly populations, medical experts take these modifications into account.

For older persons taking Contrave, customized evaluations, consistent monitoring, and dosage modifications might be required to maximize safety and effectiveness.

**2. Considerations Associated with Gender:**

**a. Being pregnant and nursing:** It is unknown if Contrave is safe to use when pregnant or nursing. There is a dearth of information on the possible dangers to a growing fetus or breastfeeding child.

It is generally not advised to use contrave when nursing. Alternative approaches to weight control are discussed by healthcare experts with nursing mothers in order to protect the health of the mother and her child.

**b. Gender Variations in the Management of Weight:** Strategies for managing weight and reactions to medicine may be influenced by gender-related characteristics. When creating individualized treatment regimens for patients with varying gender identities, medical practitioners take these issues into consideration.

Personalized strategies that take into account each person's requirements, preferences, and any gender-specific factors lead to more successful weight management outcomes.

**3. Cultural Elements:**

**a. Cultural Awareness in the Management of Weight:** Culture has a big impact on how people feel about their bodies, what they eat, and how active they are. Healthcare practitioners include cultural awareness into conversations and interventions related to weight management.

Understanding and respecting various cultural viewpoints on lifestyle, diet, and health are essential components of providing treatment that is culturally competent.

**b. Styles of Communication:** Cultural quirks affect effective communication. Diverse communication styles are used by healthcare workers to build trust and collaboration with people from various cultural backgrounds.

To improve the efficacy of weight control counseling, linguistic considerations, cultural values, and health beliefs are integrated into patient-provider interactions.

**4. Conditions Comorbid:**

**a. Mental Health Comorbidities:** When prescribing Contrave, people with psychiatric comorbidities might need special consideration. Given the medication's propensity to affect mood and behavior, examinations and cooperative management with mental health specialists are required.

Discussions about how to balance the effects on psychiatric illnesses with weight management goals are part of shared decision-making.

**b. Heart-related Conditions:** Blood pressure and heart rate are just two of the cardiovascular health consequences of contrave. People who already have cardiovascular issues need to work with cardiovascular specialists and undergo comprehensive evaluations.

Plans specifically designed to reduce cardiovascular risk are created, keeping in mind the need to strike a balance between cardiovascular safety and weight control goals.

**5. Particular Populations:**

**a. People who suffer from renal impairment:** There hasn't been enough research done on the safety and effectiveness of Contrave in those with end-stage renal disease or severe renal impairment. Individualized renal function assessments and consultation with nephrologists are essential.

For those with renal impairment, Contrave dosage adjustments or evaluation of alternate weight-management techniques may be required.

**b. People who suffer from hepatic impairment:** The metabolism of the ingredients in Contrave may be impacted by hepatic impairment. Standard procedure calls for close monitoring of liver function, with hepatic function evaluations serving as the basis for treatment plan modifications.

In order to protect patients with hepatic impairment, healthcare providers interact with specialists and take into account the possibility of hepatotoxicity.

**c. People who suffer from respiratory conditions:** Due to the possible respiratory side effects of Contrave, people who already have respiratory issues may need to be given extra attention. It is crucial to manage together with respiratory specialists.

Efficient identification and handling of such consequences are facilitated by comprehensive evaluations and close observation for respiratory indications.

**d. People who have diabetes:** The effects of contrave on glucose metabolism may affect diabetics. Adjusting antidiabetic medication, closely monitoring glucose control, and working with endocrinologists are essential.

Patients with diabetes are empowered to actively manage their condition when they receive patient education about blood glucose monitoring and possible swings in blood glucose levels.

**6. Effect on Life Quality:**

**a. Effect on the Mind:** Attempts to lose weight, especially when using drugs like Contrave, may have psychological effects. Changes in one's overall well-being, self-esteem, and body image are possible.

Healthcare practitioners understand the value of addressing the emotional components of the trip and incorporate psychological support into weight management strategies.

**b. Social Factors:** Success in managing weight is influenced by social factors, such as relationships, family dynamics, and social support networks. In order to create comprehensive and long-lasting treatment regimens, healthcare practitioners investigate these factors.

Comprehensive weight management treatments include addressing potential social barriers, incorporating family members in lifestyle changes, and promoting social support.

A wide range of characteristics are taken into account while evaluating Contrave, underscoring the need of providing individualized and patient-centered therapy. To maximize the safety and effectiveness of Contrave in a variety of individuals, healthcare practitioners manage age-specific considerations, gender-related issues, cultural nuances, concomitant conditions, and specialized populations. Comprehensive evaluations, cooperative decision-making, and continual observation are components of holistic weight control approaches that put the physical and mental health of the patient first. Healthcare providers can help ensure that each patient receiving tailored care is meeting their own requirements and circumstances by taking these special concerns into account.

# MONITORING REQUIREMENTS

Monitoring people taking Contrave entails a thorough process that takes into account many facets of their health and welfare. When it comes to performing routine examinations, lab work, and assessments to guarantee the safe and efficient use of Contrave, healthcare providers are essential. In this thorough investigation, we examine the monitoring needs related to Contrave, addressing important topics such blood testing, lifestyle tracking, mental evaluations, and cardiovascular monitoring. These factors are essential for determining possible side effects, customizing treatment regimens, and achieving the best possible weight management results.

**1. Heart-Risk Assessment:**

**a. Evaluations of Blood Pressure:** Monitoring people taking Contrave requires routine blood pressure checks. There is a chance that the medicine will raise blood pressure, however regular monitoring can help spot changes in blood pressure.

Before starting Contrave, medical personnel take baseline blood pressure readings and perform routine follow-up exams. Cardiovascular risk variables are used to define the objectives for an individual's blood pressure.

**b. Heart Rate Tracking:** Contrave may affect heart rate, so it's crucial to keep an eye out for any changes, particularly in people who already have cardiovascular disease. Continuous monitoring and baseline heart rate evaluations aid in the identification of possible cardiovascular consequences.

Based on individual risk factors and cardiovascular health, customized heart rate objectives are set. When necessary, cardiovascular specialists work with healthcare providers.

**c. Monitoring of an electrocardiogram (ECG):** Healthcare providers may occasionally think about baseline and sporadic ECG monitoring, especially for patients with underlying cardiovascular diseases. ECG evaluations assist in identifying possible modifications to heart rhythm.

More frequent ECG monitoring may be part of collaborative management with cardiologists for people who are more likely to experience cardiovascular events.

## 2. Psychiatric Evaluations:

**a. Behavioral and Emotional Tracking:** Contrave may affect behavior and mood due to its bupropion component. Frequent evaluations of behavior, mood, and emotions aid in spotting any abnormalities or side effects.

Open communication between patients and healthcare providers encourages people to disclose any behavioral issues or mood swings. It could be essential to engage in collaborative management with mental health specialists.

**b. Assessing the Risk of Suicidality:** Bupropion is recognized to carry a risk of suicidality. In-depth risk assessments are carried out by medical specialists, particularly for those with a history of depression or suicidal thoughts.

It's critical to keep an eye out for mood swings, elevated anxiety, or suicide thoughts. Managing possible dangers requires early intervention and coordination with mental health professionals.

**c. Review of Psychiatric History:** Before writing a prescription for Contrave, medical practitioners thoroughly analyze each patient's psychiatric history. Assessments for a history of eating disorders, drug use problems, and other mental health issues are part of this.

Comprehending the mental health histories of individuals facilitates customized risk evaluations and treatment strategies. Working together with mental health professionals improves the approach to care as a whole.

**3. Laboratory Examinations:**

**a. Tests for Liver Function:** Because Contrave may cause hepatotoxicity, liver function tests are performed on a regular basis. A reference point is provided by baseline examinations, and variations in liver enzyme levels can be detected through continued monitoring.

Health care providers work with patients to make sure they show up for planned liver function testing. Prompt intervention is made possible by early detection of unfavorable events connected to the liver.

**b. Monitoring Lipid Profile:** Lipid profiles may be influenced by contrave. Monitoring lipid markers, such as cholesterol levels, on a regular basis aids in determining the effect on cardiovascular risk.

Personalized lipid objectives may necessitate lifestyle changes or adaptations to lipid-lowering drugs as part of collaborative care with lipid specialists.

**c. Blood Sugar Tracking:** Blood glucose levels are regularly checked in people with diabetes or who are susceptible to the effects of glucose metabolism. Due to the risk of hypo- or hyperglycemia when using Contrave, careful glucose monitoring is necessary.

Meticulous care in conjunction with endocrinologists guarantees customized glycemic control strategies. Based on trends in blood glucose, modifications to insulin regimes or anti-diabetic drugs may be required.

**d. Tests of Renal Function:** Renal function tests may be routinely administered to those with renal insufficiency. Although the liver is the primary site of contrave metabolism, it is crucial to evaluate renal function in populations whose renal health is compromised.

A complete approach to weight management that takes renal health into consideration is ensured by collaborative management with nephrologists or renal specialists.

## 4. Tracking Lifestyle:

**a. Monitoring Body Mass Index (BMI) and Weight:** It is essential to regularly track weight and BMI in order to evaluate how well Contrave works for weight management objectives. Clinical recommendations serve as the basis for the establishment of individualized weight loss goals.

Healthcare practitioners recognize the value of slow and sustainable weight loss and offer continuing support and encouragement. Treatment strategies may need to be modified in light of each patient's unique reaction.

**b. Evaluations of Physical Activity:** Improved physical activity and other lifestyle changes are key components of weight management. Individuals are better able to monitor their progress and pinpoint areas for development when their levels of physical activity are regularly assessed.

Experts in healthcare offer advice on how to fit exercise into everyday schedules. The focus of collaborative efforts is on attainable and realistic activity goals.

**c. Nutritional monitoring and dietary counseling:** One essential element of weight management is dietary guidance. Overall success is influenced by routine evaluations of eating behaviors, nutritional intake, and adherence to dietary guidelines.

Dietitians and healthcare experts work together to provide individualized dietary regimens. Ensuring that there is adequate nutrition guarantees that weight loss is accomplished in a healthy way.

**d. Assistance in Quitting Smoking:** One of the ingredients in Contrave, bupropion, is utilized as a smoking cessation medication. Those who use Contrave to help them quit smoking and manage their weight also benefit from extra support in quitting tobacco.

Working together with experts or programs that help people quit smoking increases the efficacy of therapies. Evaluating smoking status is part of routine follow-up exams.

**5. Monitoring Adverse Events:**

**a. Reporting and Communicating with Patients:** It is advised that anyone using Contrave notify their healthcare providers as soon as possible if they experience any negative side effects or adverse events. Early detection and intervention are made easier by open communication.

Health care providers encourage people to voice any questions or concerns and offer clear advise on possible side effects. In shared decision-making, the monitoring process is actively participated in.

**b. Documentation of Adverse Events:** Healthcare practitioners systematically record adverse events that are reported, along with the type and intensity of symptoms. Precise and exhaustive record-keeping enhances the overall comprehension of a person's reaction to Contrave.

Working together with reporting systems or pharmacovigilance systems guarantees that adverse events are recorded and examined for patterns or trends.

**c. Managing Collectively with Experts:** When certain negative outcomes or difficulties occur, a collaborative management approach with experts is started. Consultations with cardiologists, endocrinologists, psychologists, and other experts may be necessary for this.

Individuals who receive multidisciplinary treatment are guaranteed to receive comprehensive support and expertise customized to meet their specific health needs.

In order to guarantee the safe and efficient use of the drug, monitoring criteria related to Contrave are crucial. Regular evaluations of test results, adverse events, psychological health, cardiovascular health, and lifestyle factors are conducted by healthcare specialists. Plans for individualized monitoring take into account treatment objectives, comorbid disorders, and individual risk factors. Working together, patients and healthcare providers promote candid dialogue, group decision-making, and a proactive strategy for resolving possible issues. Healthcare professionals prioritize the health and well-being of individuals on their weight reduction journey while contributing to the overall success of Contrave as a weight control intervention by following extensive monitoring procedures.

# GUIDANCE FOR PATIENTS

Giving people the knowledge they need to make informed decisions, encouraging reasonable expectations, and offering support for a successful weight-loss journey are all part of giving guidance for patients using Contrave. Healthcare providers are essential in helping patients through the process by addressing any obstacles, stressing lifestyle changes, and encouraging honest communication. In this in-depth investigation, we dive into detailed recommendations for patients on Contrave, including important topics such medication compliance, lifestyle adjustments, side effect control, and long-term weight maintenance techniques.

**1. Adherence to Medication:**

**a. Comprehending the Drug:** It is recommended that patients comprehend all the information about Contrave, such as its mechanism of action, active ingredients (naltrexone and bupropion), and intended use for weight management.

To make sure patients are knowledgeable about the medications they are taking, medical experts thoroughly explain everything and respond to any queries.

**b. Compliance with Recommended Dosage:** For Contrave to be effective and safe, the recommended dosage must be strictly followed. It is recommended that patients take their prescription exactly as prescribed by their doctor, without changing the amount or frequency.

It could be advised to use tools like reminder apps or medication organizers to encourage regular adherence to the specified schedule.

**c. Regular Timing:** To create a pattern, patients are advised to take Contrave at regular intervals throughout the day. This reduces the possibility of missing doses and maximizes the effects of the medication.

Experts in healthcare offer advice on incorporating Contrave into regular routines, such as taking it with meals or at particular times of the day.

## 2. Changes in Lifestyle:

**a. Nutritional Guidance:** Comprehensive nutritional counseling is a crucial component of the Contrave recommendations. Individualized nutrition regimens are given to patients based on their general health and weight loss objectives.

Working together with dietitians entails talking about balanced nutrition, portion control, and doable methods for introducing healthier options into regular meals.

**b. Physical Exercise Suggestions:** Successful weight management is stressed in relation to regular physical activity. Individual tastes and fitness levels are taken into consideration when creating individualized advice for patients on how to incorporate physical activity into their routines.

Medical practitioners help patients establish reasonable exercise objectives and gradually increase their level of activity over time.

**c. Assistance in Quitting Smoking:** For those who use Contrave to help them quit smoking and control their weight, extra support is offered to help them kick tobacco. Patients are urged to use the resources that are available to them or to participate in smoking cessation programs.

Working together with experts in quitting smoking improves the efficacy of therapies that target weight and smoking-related objectives.

**d. Interventions Behavioral:** Behavioral techniques are necessary for long-term weight loss. Patients are given advice on how to recognize and deal with behavioral tendencies that could lead to overindulgence in food or other harmful habits.

Counseling sessions may include cognitive-behavioral methods, goal-setting activities, and mindfulness exercises to improve self-awareness and encourage constructive behavioral changes.

**3. Management of Side Effects:**

**a. Recognizing Possible Adverse Effects:** Patients are made aware of both common and uncommon events that may occur while using Contrave. Patients can swiftly voice any concerns or symptoms when there is open communication.

In order to make sure patients are prepared, healthcare providers give a thorough rundown of all possible adverse effects at the initiation phase.

**b. Reporting Adverse Reactions:** It is advised that patients instantly notify their healthcare provider of any negative effects. Timely intervention and necessary modifications to the treatment plan are made easier by open and honest communication.

Healthcare providers reassure patients that safety and efficacy can be optimized by making adjustments and that managing side effects is a collaborative approach.

**c. Techniques for Handling Adverse Effects:** Patients are given practical tips on how to deal with frequent side effects including nausea and sleeplessness. To reduce discomfort, it could be advised to change one's lifestyle or the scheduling of Contrave.

Healthcare providers collaborate with patients to determine unique coping mechanisms and handle any side effect-related difficulties.

**4. Maintaining Weight Over Time:**

**a. Sustainable and Gradual Objectives:** Patients are given advice on how to develop realistic, progressive weight loss objectives. Stressing the value of reasonable expectations helps people succeed in the long run and reduces the chance of quickly gaining weight again.

Together with patients, healthcare providers set attainable goals and acknowledge each step of improvement.

**b. Maintaining Good Practices:** It is advised to maintain weight over the long run by forming healthy behaviors that are fostered during the use of Contrave. Patients are given the tools they need to keep up a healthy diet, consistent exercise, and mindfulness.

Health care providers help people maintain long-lasting lifestyle improvements by offering continuous support and direction on incorporating these practices into daily life.

**c. Observation and Succession:** Appointments for follow-up and routine monitoring are made in order to evaluate progress and handle any changing needs. During these sessions, patients are urged to actively participate by talking about any difficulties they may be facing and sharing their experiences.

During follow-up visits, collaborative goal-setting enables modifications to the treatment plan depending on individual responses and changing goals for weight management.

## 5. Psychological and Emotional Assistance:

**a. Taking Care of Emotional Eating:** Comprehensive guideline addresses eating disorders related to emotions. Patients get assistance in recognizing the emotional stimuli that lead to overeating and in creating non-food coping strategies.

It may be suggested to use behavioral therapies, therapy, and support groups to deal with the emotional aspects of weight management.

**b. Acknowledging Wins That Are Not Scale:** In order to acknowledge improvement that goes beyond the numbers on the scale, patients are urged to identify and celebrate non-scale achievements. Improvements in mood, vitality, fit of clothes, and general wellbeing are all included in this.

Healthcare providers encourage a positive outlook by emphasizing the various facets of weight management success.

**c. Check-ins for Mental Health:** The treatment of patients includes routine check-ins for mental health. Inquiries are made of patients regarding their general state of health, their stress levels, and any shifts in their emotional state.

For those managing stress, anxiety, or other mental health issues, collaborative management with mental health specialists may include extra support.

**6. Tailored Care Programs:**

**a. Use of Tailoring Contrave:** Contrave advice is tailored to each patient's particular requirements, preferences, and medical concerns. Plans for treatment are customized to maximize both efficacy and safety.
In order to ensure that treatment plans accurately represent each patient's goals and preferences, healthcare practitioners actively involve patients in shared decision-making.

**b. Honest Communication:** Throughout the course of the Contrave treatment, open communication is encouraged. It is important for patients to communicate to their healthcare provider any worries, inquiries, or changes in their health.
Frequent check-ins, whether in person or virtually, give patients the chance to talk with their healthcare team about their triumphs, struggles, and experiences.

**c. Cooperative Decision-Making:** The foundational principle of Contrave guidance is shared decision-making. Patients take an active role in choosing their course of care, establishing reasonable objectives, and modifying the plan of care in response to their unique needs.

A sense of empowerment and ownership is fostered by collaborative efforts, which improve the patient experience as a whole.

Thorough advice for Contrave users encompasses a variety of topics, including treatment planning, lifestyle adjustments, managing side effects, maintaining weight over the long term, emotional and psychological support, and medication adherence. When it comes to providing patients with the information and resources they need to successfully control their weight, healthcare providers are essential. Healthcare professionals enhance the general well-being of people on their journey to reaching and maintaining a healthier weight by encouraging open communication, establishing reasonable expectations, and offering continuous support.

# LIFESTYLE RECOMMENDATIONS

A key component of effective weight management is the implementation of lifestyle recommendations, which support behavioral techniques, dietary adjustments, and medication use. Personalized lifestyle advice promotes long-term weight loss, better general health, and increased wellbeing. We explore a wide range of lifestyle advice in this thorough investigation, covering things like stress management, physical activity, mindful practices, sleep hygiene, and nutrition.

**1. Food**

**a. A well-rounded diet:** Stress the value of eating a varied, nutrient-dense diet that is balanced. To ensure that you are getting enough vitamins and minerals, promote the consumption of fruits, vegetables, lean proteins, whole grains, and healthy fats.

Work together with qualified dietitians to create customized meal plans that satisfy each person's dietary requirements and support weight loss objectives.

**b. Control of Portion:** Promote portion control as a vital element of a balanced diet. Teach people how to identify the right portion sizes in order to reduce overindulgence and encourage mindful eating.

Provide visual signals or tools to help with portion estimate so that people can learn how to prepare balanced meals.

**c. Drinking plenty of water:** Emphasize the value of drinking water to stay properly hydrated throughout the day. In addition to helping with digestion and general health, hydration can also increase feelings of fullness.

Urge people to stick to drinking water as their main beverage and to avoid consuming too many sugar-filled drinks, which can add extra calories.

**d. Optimal Timing for Meals:** To encourage a regular eating routine, set up regular meal times. To control hunger and preserve energy levels, encourage people to eat organized meals and snacks at regular intervals.

Work together to create meals that complement daily schedules, taking individual tastes, physical activity levels, and work schedules into account.

**e. Conscious Eating Techniques:** Practice mindful eating to increase your awareness of your body's signals of hunger and fullness. Urge people to pay attention to their bodies' cues, enjoy every bite, and eat in silence.

Incorporate mindfulness exercises to promote a healthy connection with eating, such as gratitude exercises or mindful breathing.

**2. Engaging in Exercise:**

**a. Tailored Fitness Programs:** Create customized training regimens that take into account each person's preferences, degree of fitness, and any underlying medical issues. Work together with fitness experts to develop customized programs that support weight loss objectives.

To enhance general fitness, encourage a mix of strength training, flexibility training, and aerobic activities.

**b. Gradual Advancement:** Stress the value of increasing physical activity gradually. To reduce the risk of injury and improve adherence to long-term fitness regimens, discourage overindulgent exercise or sudden increases in intensity.

Encourage them to set reasonable fitness objectives and modify their workout plans as their strength and endurance increase.

**c. Continuity:** Emphasize how important consistency is to sustaining an active lifestyle. Engaging in consistent and regular physical activity promotes cardiovascular health, weight management, and general well-being.

Help people incorporate physical activity into their everyday routines by walking or biking to work, using the stairs, or participating in enjoyable hobbies.

**d. Diverse Exercise Methods:** To keep things interesting and promote general fitness, try incorporating different types of exercise. To keep physical activity interesting, try out new things like swimming, cycling, yoga, or group classes.

Work together with fitness experts to teach a variety of workouts that focus on different muscle groups and enhance functional fitness in general.

**e. After-Workout Recovery:** Emphasize the significance of recuperating from activity by getting enough rest, being hydrated, and stretching. Stress the importance of recuperation in lowering the risk of injury, preventing tiredness, and maintaining muscular health.

Give advice on adding rest days to the workout regimen and using recovery techniques like foam rolling or light stretching.

## 3. Suitable Sleep Position:

**a. Regular Sleep Schedule:** Encourage adherence to a regular sleep pattern in order to maintain overall health and balance circadian rhythms. Encourage people to wake up and go to bed at the same hour every day, including on the weekends.

Work together with sleep professionals to treat any disturbances or problems that could affect the quality of your sleep.

**b. Establish a Setting That Encourages Sleep:** Give advice on how to create a setting that encourages sleep. This entails avoiding using electronics right before bed and maintaining a cool, dark, and quiet bedroom.

Talk about the significance of creating a pre-sleep routine, such reading a book or using relaxation techniques, to tell the body that it's time to shut down.

**c. Minimize Electronics Before Sleep:** Advise against using stimulants right before bed, such as nicotine or coffee. These drugs may cause sleep cycles to be disturbed and may make it difficult to fall asleep.

Work together with each person to create plans for cutting back on or giving up stimulants in the hours before bed.

**d. Frequent Exercise:** Encourage frequent exercise as a way to improve the quality of your sleep. Exercise of a moderate level during the day can lengthen and increase the effectiveness of sleep.

Work with folks to choose appropriate times for physical activity that don't interfere with their sleep patterns and fit into their daily schedules.

**e. Techniques for Stress Management:** To reduce stress before bed, introduce stress management strategies. Before going to bed, people can relax with techniques including progressive muscular relaxation, deep breathing, and mindfulness meditation.

Work together with mental health specialists to address underlying issues that could affect your general wellbeing and ability to sleep.

**4. Handling Stress:**

**a. Determine Your Stress Triggers:** Help people pinpoint the sources of stress in their life. Comprehending the origins of stress facilitates focused interventions and the creation of adaptive mechanisms.

Work together with counselors or psychologists to examine stressors associated with relationships, the workplace, or personal struggles.

**b. Effective Time Management:** Promote efficient time management to lessen overwhelming emotions. Urge people to prioritize their work, make realistic goals, and divide more difficult tasks into smaller, more doable ones.

Work together to create calendars or timetables that facilitate effective time management for people.

**c. Methods of Relaxation:** In order to deal with sudden tension, teach relaxation methods. Methods including gradual muscle relaxation, deep breathing, and guided visualization can help lower the body's and mind's reaction to stress.

Work together with mental health specialists to incorporate relaxation methods into comprehensive stress-reduction strategies.

**d. Engaging in Physical Activity to Reduce Stress:** Emphasize the benefits of exercise as a potent stress reducer. Frequent physical activity can lower cortisol levels, release endorphins, and enhance happiness.

Work together with fitness experts to create workout plans that concentrate on stress management.

**e. Look for Social Assistance:** Urge them to look for social support as a way to cope with stress. Having a support network and solid social relationships can help during trying times by offering both practical and emotional support.

Work together to find people who already have support systems in place or look into ways to meet people who share your interests through community events or support organizations.

**5. Conscious Behavior:**

**a. Consciously Consuming Food:** Encourage the mindful eating technique to raise awareness of satiety, eating patterns, and meal selections. Urge them to eat gently, enjoy every piece, and pay heed to their bodies' signals of hunger and fullness.

Work with dietitians to integrate mindfulness practices into nutrition counseling sessions to promote a purposeful and positive eating strategy.

**b. Meditation with mindfulness:** Incorporate mindfulness meditation into your everyday routine to build stress reduction and present-moment awareness. People can adopt a regular meditation regimen with the help of mindfulness apps or guided meditation sessions.

Work together with mental health specialists or mindfulness practitioners to offer tools and advice on bringing mindfulness into everyday life.

**c. Exercises for Gratitude:** Encourage the practice of gratitude as a means of developing an optimistic outlook. Encourage people to write down their daily blessings in a gratitude notebook.

Work together with psychologists or counselors to investigate the role that thankfulness practices have in mental health in general.

**d. Awareness of Breath:** Teach breathing exercises to improve concentration and relaxation. Basic breathing techniques like box breathing and diaphragmatic breathing are simple enough to adopt into daily routines.

Work together with fitness experts or mindfulness practitioners to incorporate breathing exercises or mindfulness techniques into your workout regimens.

**e. Happy Occasions:** Encourage participation in happy activities that make you feel fulfilled and content. Finding things to be happy about and doing them on a daily basis improves one's general state of wellbeing.

Work together with people to discover activities, pastimes, or artistic endeavors that complement their passions and support a healthy way of life.

Thorough lifestyle suggestions are essential for helping people on their weight management path. Healthcare practitioners help people create holistic and long-lasting lifestyle improvements by addressing nutrition, exercise, sleep hygiene, stress management, and the incorporation of mindful practices. Individuals are empowered to develop healthy habits that go beyond weight reduction through tailored advice, interdisciplinary professional teamwork, and continuous support, which promotes improved overall health and well-being.

# FREQUENTLY ASKED QUESTIONS (FAQS)

Frequently Asked Questions (FAQs) are an important source of information for those looking to learn more about Contrave. These frequently asked questions (FAQs) cover a wide range of subjects and provide answers to frequently asked questions about the medication's intended use, side effects, precautions, and other pertinent information. This thorough guide seeks to help people make knowledgeable decisions regarding Contrave by offering thorough and educational answers to often asked issues.

**1. What does Contrave mean, and why is it used?**
A prescription drug called Contrave is intended to help adults control their weight. Bupropion and naltrexone are the two active components combined. While naltrexone is used to treat addiction, it may also assist regulate weight by regulating the brain's reward system. Bupropion is an antidepressant that may do so by affecting specific neurotransmitters. When used in conjunction with a lower-calorie diet and greater physical exercise, Contrave is intended to assist people in reaching and maintaining weight loss.

**2. How Does Contrave Help in Losing Weight?**
Bupropion and naltrexone, the two active chemicals in Contrave, work together to produce its desired effects. Because bupropion alters neurotransmitters in the brain, it may cause an increase in energy expenditure and a decrease in hunger. Conversely, naltrexone may affect the brain's reward system, so lessening the reinforcing benefits of eating. When combined, these systems seek to help people reduce weight by assisting them in managing their food intake and choosing better lifestyle options.

**3. What Constitutes Contrave's Active Ingredients?**
Naltrexone hydrochloride and bupropion hydrochloride are the active components in Contrave. Naltrexone is an opioid receptor antagonist, and bupropion is an atypical antidepressant. It is believed that these two elements working together will improve weight control.

**4. What Constituents of Contrave Are Inactive?**
Fillers, binders, and coloring agents are a few examples of the inactive substances in Contrave. These inactive components are intended to support the medication's stability and formulation. Individuals with known allergies or sensitivities to certain compounds should refer to the package insert

of the drug or their healthcare professional for comprehensive information, since specific inactive ingredients may differ.

## 5. What Sets Contrave Apart from Other Weight Loss Drugs?

Contrave's special mix of bupropion and naltrexone sets it apart from other weight-loss drugs. Contrave's mode of action involves both the central nervous system and the brain's reward system, whereas some weight reduction drugs concentrate on suppressing hunger or inhibiting fat absorption. The selection of a weight loss medicine is influenced by various aspects, including the patient's health situation and treatment objectives. Each medication has a unique combination of advantages and possible adverse effects.

## 6. Who Qualifies as a Contrave Candidate?

Adults who have a body mass index (BMI) of 30 or higher, or a BMI of 27 or higher with at least one weight-related medical problem, such as high blood pressure or type 2 diabetes, are usually prescribed Contrave. It's crucial that people speak with their healthcare professional to find out if Contrave is a good fit for them given their unique health situation and weight loss objectives.

**7. What is the Recommended Dosage for Contrave and How is it Administered?**

Contrave is typically taken orally, though other dosages may be advised. One tablet taken in the morning is usually the starting dose, which is progressively increased to two tablets in the morning and two tablets in the evening. Individual responses and tolerability are taken into consideration when adjusting the dosage. It's critical to adhere to the recommended dosage and any further guidelines the healthcare practitioner may have offered.

**8. Contrave: Is It Safe? What Aspects of Safety Are There?**

Like any drug, contrave has advantages and disadvantages. The danger of elevated blood pressure, the possibility of seizures (particularly in those with a history of eating problems or seizures), and the possibility of suicidal thoughts are among the safety concerns (given the presence of bupropion). Healthcare professionals make sure Contrave is safe and appropriate for usage by thoroughly evaluating a patient's medical history, current conditions, and any contraindications before prescribing it.

**9. What Are Contrave's Typical Side Effects?**

Nausea, constipation, headaches, vomiting, dizziness, sleeplessness, and dry mouth are common adverse effects of Contrave. People must notify their healthcare professional as soon as they experience any negative effects. These adverse effects might vary in degree and are not always felt by the same person. In order to manage side effects and decide on the best course of action, which may involve changing dosages or implementing other interventions, healthcare providers collaborate with patients.

## 10. Do Serious Adverse Reactions Occur With Contrave?

Although Contrave is generally well tolerated, there is a chance of major adverse effects. A higher chance of suicidal thoughts, seizures, elevated blood pressure, liver damage, and allergic responses are a few of these. People must notify their healthcare professional right away if they have any unsettling side effects or symptoms. Healthcare professionals carefully review a patient's medical history and look for any potential hazards before prescribing Contrave.

## 11. Does Contrave Mix with Other Prescription Drugs?

It is important for people to provide a detailed list of all the drugs, vitamins, and herbal products they are taking because Contrave can interact with other prescriptions. Contrave may interact negatively with some drugs, such as monoamine oxidase inhibitors (MAOIs). Before administering Contrave, medical professionals thoroughly consider any possible drug interactions and modify treatment regimens as necessary.

## 12. Does the Use of Contrave Affect Mental Health?

Bupropion is an antidepressant included in Contrave that may have an impact on mood. While for some people it can have a favorable impact on their mood, there is a chance that it will exacerbate suicide thoughts, especially during the early phases of treatment. When using Contrave, medical professionals keep a close eye on patients' mental health, and those who have a history of mental health issues could need more care and support.

## 13. Is It Safe to Take Contrave While Breastfeeding or During Pregnancy?

Contrave's safety during pregnancy and lactation has not been proven, hence using it during these times is usually not advised. Those who are pregnant or intend to become pregnant should talk to their healthcare physician about alternate weight management techniques. Similarly, those who are nursing should get advice from their healthcare professional regarding whether to stop nursing or pursue other methods for managing their weight.

**14. For How Long Is Contrave Safe to Take? For Long-Term Use Only?**

The length of time a patient uses Contrave depends on their personal weight management objectives and the doctor's evaluation. While some people may use Contrave for longer-term maintenance, others may use it for a set amount of time to reach their initial weight loss goals. Healthcare professionals work with patients to identify the ideal period of Contrave use by routinely monitoring side effects, tracking progress, and collaborating with them.

**15. Is Contrave Effective for Quitting Smoking?**

Indeed, one of Contrave's main chemicals, bupropion, is also utilized as a smoking cessation aid. People who use Contrave to control their weight may also benefit from support in quitting smoking. When prescribing Contrave for more than one purpose, however, medical professionals take into account the preferences and specific health factors of each patient.

**16. What Is the Expected Weight Loss with Contrave?**

Different people may lose different amounts of weight while using Contrave. According to clinical trials, those who use Contrave may, on average, lose a little weight in comparison to people who use a placebo. The real amount of weight reduction is determined by a number of variables, including genetics, individual metabolism, and following food and lifestyle guidelines. Healthcare professionals assist patients in setting reasonable weight loss objectives and track their advancement over time.

**17. What Takes Place if a Contrave Dose Is Missed?**

A person should take their missed dose of Contrave as soon as they remember. They should, however, forego the missed dose and resume the regular dosing plan if the time for the next scheduled dose is approaching. It is not advised to double up on dosages to make up for a missed one. If someone needs advice on their medication regimen or has questions regarding missed doses, they should get in touch with their healthcare professional.

**18. Is it Possible to Combine Contrave with Other Weight Loss Techniques?**

Yes, doctors frequently prescribe Contrave in addition to lower-calorie diets and increased physical activity to help patients lose weight. When combined with comprehensive lifestyle changes, Contrave becomes even more effective in aiding in weight loss. Healthcare professionals collaborate with patients to create individualized weight-management programs that include several approaches for the best outcomes.

**19. When taking Contrave, how often should people follow up with their healthcare provider?**
Keeping up with follow-up appointments with doctors is crucial when using Contrave. Follow-up appointments vary in frequency, although they are usually more frequent during the first phases of treatment. During these consultations, medical professionals can evaluate side effects, track progress, and alter the treatment plan as needed. Participants are urged to actively engage in these follow-up appointments by disclosing any changes in their health or any worries they may have about using Contrave.

**20. Can You Continue Losing Weight After Stopping Contrave?**
After stopping Contrave, maintaining weight loss depends on a number of things, one of which is

continuing to lead a healthy lifestyle. Contrave is a weight-loss help, but prolonged dietary adjustments, consistent exercise, and other lifestyle changes are necessary for long-term success. Healthcare professionals emphasize the value of keeping healthy practices while working with patients to establish strategies for maintaining weight loss even after stopping Contrave.

The Contrave Frequently Asked Questions (FAQs) offer insightful information regarding the drug's intended use, safety precautions, and a range of topics related to its influence on weight management. These thorough answers are meant to help people make educated decisions regarding Contrave, but they also stress how crucial it is to work together with healthcare professionals to receive individualized advice and assistance. People who are thinking about using Contrave or who are already using it are advised to speak with their healthcare providers for personalized guidance based on their individual health profiles and weight loss objectives.

# CONCLUSION

The thorough examination of Contrave, in summary, demonstrates a complex strategy for managing weight. It covers a wide range of topics, including its intended use, active and inactive ingredients, mechanisms of action, medical applications, patient eligibility requirements, suggested dosage, administration guidelines, efficacy studies, safety concerns, adverse reactions, and other crucial elements. The goal of this in-depth analysis is to give patients and medical professionals a better understanding of Contrave, enabling them to make informed decisions and promote safe and efficient use.

As a prescription drug, Contrave is at the nexus of weight control and obesity, the intricate field of weight and pharmaceutical innovation. Its major goal is to help adults lose weight and keep it off. It also provides a therapeutic option for those who have a body mass index (BMI) of 30 or higher, or a BMI of 27 or higher and are dealing with medical concerns related to their weight. The combination of naltrexone and bupropion, the active components, affects neurotransmitters and the brain's reward system, which helps regulate hunger and promotes better lifestyle choices.

Together, the active components naltrexone hydrochloride and bupropion hydrochloride address various facets of weight management. As bupropion affects neurotransmitters, it may decrease appetite and increase energy expenditure; on the other hand, naltrexone may affect the brain's reward system, which could lessen the reinforcement that food provides. Contrave stands apart from other weight-loss drugs due to this special mix; each drug has its own advantages, working principles, and possible drawbacks.

Oral ingestion of the prescription is required, and the dosage should be gradually increased to the entire specified amount over time. Eligibility for patients is established by BMI and related medical issues; healthcare providers carefully review each patient's profile to make sure they are a good fit. The dosage recommendation is based on the reaction and tolerance of each individual, with a focus on the significance of following prescribed schedules.

Clinical studies attest to Contrave's effectiveness and show that, when paired with a lower-calorie diet and more exercise, it may help with weight loss. The drug's effects go beyond what is seen on the outside; it can help those who want to stop smoking. This multifunctionality, however, emphasizes how crucial it is to take into account a number of variables, including mental health, in the entire treatment strategy.

When using Contrave, safety must always come first. Common side effects like nausea and sleeplessness are possible, as well as more severe ones like elevated blood pressure and a higher chance of seizures. The medicine needs to be closely monitored, particularly in people who already have health issues. Healthcare professionals are essential in determining the risk-benefit profile of each patient.

Comprehending the safety profile of the medication requires a thorough investigation of side effects, both mild and severe. In order to navigate these possible consequences, patients and healthcare providers must communicate openly and collaboratively to address any obstacles that may come up throughout therapy.

Contrave is not a one-size-fits-all medication; rather, patient eligibility must be carefully considered, dosage recommendations must be followed, and continuous safety and efficacy monitoring is necessary. Healthcare providers are able to customize treatment regimens to meet the needs of each patient by using patient eligibility criteria that take into account variables including BMI, pre-existing medical problems, and contraindications.

The usefulness of Contrave is informed by recommended dosage, administration recommendations, and efficacy studies taken together. These elements support the medication's overall efficacy by giving patients and medical practitioners a defined framework for navigating the challenges of weight management.

The effects of the medication go beyond the physical and also affect emotional and mental wellness. Due to its antidepressant nature, Contrave should be used with caution in order to avoid negative effects on mood or an increased risk of suicide ideation. A comprehensive approach to care must be ensured through coordination with mental health providers and mental health check-ins.

There is more to Contrave's journey from prescription to successful weight management than merely popping a pill. It requires a dedication to dietary adjustments, greater physical exercise, and the development of mindful practices, among other lifestyle changes. A key component of Contrave's all-encompassing strategy is its lifestyle suggestions, which support long-term weight loss, better general health, and increased wellbeing.

Effective weight control is facilitated by the adoption of healthy behaviors, such as a balanced diet, consistent exercise, and enough sleep. Changing one's lifestyle goes hand in hand with taking Contrave; together, they create a synergistic approach that goes beyond the drug's initial effects. Under the direction of medical specialists, individualized treatment plans enable people to make long-lasting adjustments and sustain a healthier weight in the long run.

Contrave's all-encompassing influence reaches the emotional and psychological domains in addition to the physical. The medication's holistic approach includes addressing emotional eating, encouraging a good mindset, and recognizing non-scale triumphs. Contrave's patient advice incorporates emotional well-being into its core principles, acknowledging the connection between mental and physical health.

Beyond just writing a prescription, patient assistance includes arming people with knowledge that is critical to their health, encouraging reasonable expectations, and offering encouragement to achieve and maintain a healthy weight. A patient-centered strategy incorporates medication adherence, lifestyle adjustments, side effect control, and long-term weight maintenance measures. In order to help patients through the process, healthcare providers are essential in highlighting the value of candid communication and group decision-making.

Requirements for monitoring Contrave highlight the dedication to guaranteeing the drug is used safely and effectively. To provide a complete picture of an individual's reaction, regular evaluations of cardiovascular health, mental health, laboratory parameters, lifestyle factors, and adverse events are necessary. Working together, patients and healthcare providers promote candid dialogue, group decision-making, and a pro-active strategy for resolving possible issues.

Patients are given advice that goes beyond the short-term course of treatment and includes long-term weight maintenance techniques. The cornerstones of successful weight management are the continuation of good behaviors, gradual and sustainable objectives, and constant monitoring and follow-up. A comprehensive and long-lasting approach to health and well-being includes regular check-ins with mental health providers, addressing emotional eating, and celebrating achievement beyond the scale.

The recommendations for Contrave's impact on lifestyle also include good eating, exercise, good sleep hygiene, stress reduction, and thoughtful activities. The effects of the drug are enhanced by customized lifestyle advice, which advance general health and wellbeing. These suggestions encourage a whole-life lifestyle by enabling people to take up healthy practices that go beyond losing weight.

If someone is looking for information about Contrave, the Frequently Asked Questions (FAQs) are a great resource. These frequently asked questions (FAQs) cover a wide range of subjects and provide answers to frequently asked questions about the medication's intended use, side effects, precautions, and other pertinent information. This thorough guide seeks to help people make knowledgeable decisions regarding Contrave by offering thorough and educational answers to often asked issues.

Contrave shows itself to be more than just a medicine for weight loss; it is an all-encompassing strategy for health and wellbeing. Contrave navigates the complex world of weight control with ease, providing everything from its mechanism and goal to patient counsel, lifestyle suggestions, and frequently asked questions. It necessitates collaboration between patients and medical specialists, encouraging candid dialogue, group decision making, and a dedication to long-term health.

The path taken by Contrave has been dynamic, influenced by continuing research, clinical discoveries, and the growing body of knowledge regarding obesity and weight control. When people start taking Contrave, they are not just accepting a prescription; they are also joining forces to reach and stay at a healthier weight. This exploration's conclusion signifies a journey rather than a point of completion, as people and medical professionals work together to traverse the challenges of weight control in order to promote resilience, long-term health, and overall well-being.

Manufactured by Amazon.ca
Bolton, ON